EXECUTIVE SUMMARY

Americans living in rural areas face a shortage of primary care physicians and specialists, and often must travel large distances to obtain medical care. The increasing cost of providing health care and the demands of an aging population also put pressures on rural health care providers, many of which struggle to keep their doors open.

The Federal Communications Commission (Commission or FCC) has implemented the statutory mandate for universal service by, among other things, creating the Rural Health Care (RHC) program to improve access to communications services for eligible health care providers. In recent years, broadband has become increasingly vital to the effective delivery of health care, and it can be uniquely transformative in rural areas, where distance poses a substantial challenge. In recognition of this, the Commission in 2006 launched the Rural Health Care Pilot Program (Pilot Program), which awarded 69 projects one-time funding for a defined period of time (a total of $418 million) to cover up to 85 percent of the cost of construction and deployment of broadband networks that connect participating health care providers in rural and urban areas. The Pilot Program currently supports 50 active projects in 38 states (the "Pilot projects") and the territories of Guam, American Samoa and the Northern Mariana Islands. Many of the Pilot broadband networks have been established and are now delivering the benefits of telemedicine and other telehealth applications to their patients.

In creating the Pilot Program, the Commission sought to harness the potential of broadband health care provider networks to improve the quality and reduce the cost of health care in rural areas, while drawing on that experience to inform the redesign of its permanent RHC program. A key component of any pilot program is the opportunity to evaluate what has been learned and how those experiences can inform future work – in this case, the Commission's ongoing oversight and management of its universal service programs. This Staff Report provides an evaluation of the successes and challenges of the Pilot projects to date. The Report describes the projects, their broadband networks, and the financial and telehealth benefits generated by their broadband connectivity. The Report presents data through January 31, 2012, except where otherwise noted.

This Report also summarizes key observations from the Pilot Program, to assist the Commission as it considers potential changes to the permanent rural health care program. In the 2010 *Notice of Proposed Rulemaking* (*NPRM*), the Commission proposed a number of changes to improve access to broadband services and broadband infrastructure for health care providers, building on the recommendations of the 2010 *National Broadband Plan*.

As is clear from this Report, the Pilot Program provides fertile ground to help the Commission determine how best to reform the existing rural health care program, which provides ongoing support for telecommunications and Internet access services. The following are key facts, benefits, and lessons of the Pilot Program to date:

Key Facts About the Pilot Program:

- As of January 2012, 2,107 health care providers were on target to receive $217 million in universal service support through the Pilot Program (an average of about $100,000 per health care provider over the award period).

- Projects range in size from fewer than ten to over 150 health care provider sites; about a third of the projects each have over 50 health care provider sites receiving support through the Pilot Program.

- The five largest projects are statewide networks located in California, Colorado, Oregon, South Carolina, and West Virginia. So far, these networks are on target to receive funding to connect over 800 health care providers.

- Forty-four of 50 projects that receive Pilot Program support include urban health care providers. Approximately 35 percent of all health care providers that had received funding commitments in the Pilot Program as of January 2012 were classified as urban, or 733 of the 2,107 total.

- Leaders of Pilot projects often come from large medical institutions and universities, which frequently are located in urban areas. The urban health care providers often serve as hubs for the network, and as such receive support for the equipment that enables the entire network to operate.

- Pilot project participants purchase higher bandwidth connections than do participants in the Commission's existing program, which defrays the cost of telecommunications and Internet access services for health care providers in rural areas. Most Pilot Project participants purchase 10 Mbps or faster connections, which are much faster than the connections that typically are purchased in the permanent RHC Program, the vast majority of which are 3 Mbps or less.

- The majority of Pilot projects choose to purchase broadband services from commercial providers rather than construct and own their own broadband networks.

Key Benefits of the Pilot Program. Support through the Pilot Program has helped health care providers obtain broadband capability to implement telemedicine and telehealth applications. Telemedicine and telehealth applications improve the quality of health care delivered to patients in rural areas, generate savings in the cost of providing health care, and reduce the time and expense associated with travel to distant locations to receive or provide care. Although many Pilot projects are still assembling their networks, the projects have already demonstrated how broadband health care networks can significantly improve the quality and reduce the cost of providing health care in rural areas. For example:

- The Palmetto State Providers Network, located in South Carolina, reports that it has saved $18 million dollars in Medicaid costs over 18 months as a result of its tele-psychiatry program. Psychiatric consults are now available 24/7. Previously, patients would take up valuable health care provider time and resources by having to wait for days to receive psychiatric consults.

- In Pennsylvania, Geisinger Health System notes that its network provides tele-stroke services for neurology patients within minutes as opposed to hours. Given that "time is brain" for stroke victims, instant access to specialized care can be life-saving.

- All of Geisinger's Pilot project health care providers are members of a Health Information Exchange that links 53 hospitals and 9,000 physicians, and they have adopted, implemented, upgraded, or successfully demonstrated the use of certified Electronic Health Record technology.

- In South Dakota, the Heartland Unified Broadband Network (HUBNet) estimates that hospitals in its network have saved $1.2 million in transfer expenses over a 30-month period, following the implementation of electronic Intensive Care Unit (e-ICU) services. HUBNet also has dropped the average number of days patients spend in ICU, thereby reducing costs, and has reduced the number of patient transfers to other hospitals.

- Pennsylvania Mountains Healthcare Alliance's network has reduced the turnaround time on X-ray readings from 20 to 7 minutes.

- Continuing medical education provides rural providers with increased learning opportunities and reduces their sense of medical isolation. For example, rural sites participating in the Iowa Rural Health Telecommunications Program report that the network and the telemedicine services provided over it have enhanced physician satisfaction and collegial support.

Key Lessons Learned from the Pilot Program. This report also summarizes key observations drawn from successful Pilot Programs. These observations include:

- *Broadband health care networks improve the quality and reduce the cost of delivering health care in rural areas.* Broadband makes possible the use of telemedicine to improve health care delivery in rural areas. In addition to delivering needed medical care to patients in remote locations, telemedicine lowers the cost of providing health care, reduces travel time and expense for patients, providers and doctors, and brings needed revenue to endangered rural clinics and hospitals. Broadband networks also facilitate other important telehealth applications – such as the transmission of medical images, exchange of electronic health records, remote consultations with specialists, and training of rural medical personnel.

- *Consortium applications are more efficient.* Consortium applications save time and money for applicants and for the Universal Service Administrative Company (USAC), which administers rural health care programs under the Commission's direction. Consortium applications allow health care providers to spread administrative, network design, and other costs over a large number of entities. They also enable smaller health care providers to take advantage of the expertise and resources of larger providers, and they foster the formation of coordinated networks of health care providers.

- *Bulk buying plus competitive bidding is a powerful combination.* Consortium purchasing by a large number of geographically dispersed sites, coupled with competitive bidding, can yield higher bandwidth, lower prices, and better service quality for the Pilot projects.

- *Urban sites are key members of rural health care provider networks.* As the Western New York Pilot project put it, without its urban partners it would be "building a road to nowhere." Broadband networks often bring to patients in rural areas the additional medical expertise, creativity, technical know-how, and innovation available in large urban medical centers. The leadership, technical and medical expertise, and administrative resources provided by urban health care providers also have proved central to the success of many Pilot projects.

- *Most health care providers do not have the technical expertise to manage broadband networks and do not want to own such networks.* The majority of Pilot projects have created successful broadband networks by purchasing broadband services from a third party, rather than constructing and owning their own broadband facilities. Mechanisms such as long-term leases, prepaid leases, and indefeasible rights of use of facilities for specified period of time (IRUs) help many projects obtain the bandwidth and service quality they needed.

- *Funding challenges remain for rural health care providers.* Rural health care providers operate on a thin margin, or in the red, and universal service support helps many to access the benefits of broadband.

TABLE OF CONTENTS

I.   INTRODUCTION

1. The Wireline Competition Bureau (Bureau) staff has prepared this Staff Report (Report) to assist the Federal Communications Commission in considering reforms to the Rural Health Care (RHC) support mechanism and in developing sound evaluation plans for any new programs. The Report both describes and extracts lessons from the Commission's Rural Health Care Pilot Program (Pilot Program),

which provides universal service support to extend broadband networks for health care providers (HCPs).[1] As discussed more fully below, the Report provides concrete data regarding the efficacy of broadband networks in delivering health care to rural America. The Report also provides extensive information that will assist the Commission in addressing the recommendations of the U.S. Government Accountability Office (GAO) in its November 2010 report on the Rural Health Care program.[2] The Report presents data through January 31, 2012, except where otherwise noted.

2.   The Report draws on the experiences of the Pilot projects selected in 2007: where they are now, what has worked, what has been challenging, what their broadband networks look like, and what telehealth benefits and cost savings they have realized. In order to prepare this Report, the staff spoke with a number of Pilot projects located throughout the country, which are of various sizes and at various stages of implementation. The staff also reviewed quarterly reports submitted by the Pilot projects to the Commission and data submitted by the Pilot projects at various stages of the funding process to the Universal Service Administrative Company (USAC), the entity that performs the day-to-day administration of the program under Commission oversight. The Report also reports on USAC's experience with the Pilot Program. USAC has provided the Commission with its own observations about the Pilot Program, as well as summaries of site visits to Pilot projects, data, and an informal assessment of the needs of rural health care providers. Because USAC is the front-line interface with the Pilot projects, USAC's insights have been particularly valuable in the preparation of this Report.[3]

3.   Many of the Pilot projects are still in the process of securing final funding commitments and implementing their networks, and so this Report can only provide a snapshot of the status of the various projects at a specific point in time (generally as of January 31, 2012, in this Report).[4] Nevertheless, many Pilot projects have already demonstrated the enormous benefits that broadband networks can bring for patients in rural areas. They have employed sophisticated telemedicine and other health IT applications over their networks, and many have begun to realize cost savings for the health care services they provide to rural Americans.[5]

4.   These benefits realized by the Pilot projects thus far fulfill one of the Commission's two goals in creating the Pilot Program: "to bring the benefits of innovative telehealth and, in particular,

---

[1] *See Rural Health Care Support Mechanism*, WC Docket No. 02-60, Order, 21 FCC Rcd 11111 (2006) (*2006 Pilot Program Order*); *Rural Health Care Support Mechanism*, WC Docket No. 02-60, Report and Order, 22 FCC Rcd 20360 (2007) (*2007 Pilot Program Selection Order*). The Commission opened participation in the Pilot Program to all eligible public and non-profit health care providers to promote the "goal of stimulating the deployment of innovative telehealth networks that will link rural health care facilities to urban health care facilities and provide telemedicine services to rural communities." *2007 Pilot Program Selection Order*, 22 FCC Rcd at 20421, para. 120.

[2] U.S. Gov't Accountability Office, FCC's Performance Management Weaknesses Could Jeopardize Proposed Reforms of the Rural Health Care Program GAO 11-27 (Nov. 2010) (*GAO Report*), *available at* http://www.gao.gov/products/GAO-11-27 (last visited Mar. 1, 2012). The *GAO Report* recommended, among other things, that the Commission assess the communications needs of rural health care providers; consult with USAC and other agencies and associations representing rural health care providers; develop effective goals, performance measures, and performance evaluation plans for current and future rural health care programs; and clearly articulate rules governing any new programs. *Id.* at 56-57.

[3] Appendix E lists the *ex parte* submissions that were used in the preparation of this Report, including submissions from the Pilot projects, USAC, and other interested parties.

[4] Most of the aggregate data used in this Report is provided as of January 31, 2012. The final deadline for submission of funding commitment requests by Pilot projects was June 30, 2012. USAC is still in the process of reviewing those requests, and will be in a position to update the data once that process is concluded later this year.

[5] *See infra* Section IV.

telemedicine services to those areas of the country where the need for those benefits is most acute."[6] The other goal of the Commission was that the Pilot Program would "lay the foundation for a future rulemaking that w[ould] explore permanent rules to enhance access to advanced services for public and non-profit health care providers" and would provide "useful information as to the feasibility of revising the Commission's current RHC rules in a manner that best achieves the objectives set forth by Congress."[7] With respect to this second goal, this Report provides analysis useful to the Commission as it considers reforms to the rural health care support mechanism to harness the potential of broadband to improve the quality and lower the cost of providing health care in rural areas across the country.[8]

5. In the years since the Commission outlined its goals for the Pilot Program, it has continued to recognize that broadband can play an important role in the transformation of health care in the 21st century, and that access to broadband is not fully realized today in all parts of the country. The Commission said in its March 16, 2010 Joint Statement on Broadband that "ubiquitous and affordable broadband can unlock vast new opportunities for Americans, in communities large and small, with respect to . . . health care delivery."[9] Additionally, the National Broadband Plan, also released on March 16, 2010, emphasized the importance of ensuring "sufficient connectivity for health care delivery locations."[10]

6. During the same time period, developments in health information technology (Health IT),[11] particularly in telehealth,[12] telemedicine,[13] and the exchange of electronic health records (EHRs),[14] have

---

[6] *2006 Pilot Program Order*, 21 FCC Rcd at 11111, para. 1.

[7] *Id.* at 11112, para. 4.

[8] *Rural Health Care Support Mechanism,* WC Docket No. 02-60, Notice of Proposed Rulemaking, 25 FCC Rcd 9371, 9373, para. 3 (2010) (*2010 NPRM or NPRM*).

[9] *Joint Statement on Broadband*, GN Docket No. 10-66, Joint Statement on Broadband, 25 FCC Rcd 3420, para. 3 (rel. Mar. 16, 2010).

[10] The National Broadband Plan recommended, among other things, that the Commission reform the RHC program by replacing the existing Internet Access Fund with a Health Care Broadband Access Fund and establishing a Health Care Broadband Infrastructure Fund to provide support for network deployment to health care delivery locations where existing networks are insufficient. Federal Communications Commission, Connecting America: The National Broadband Plan, at 200 (rel. Mar. 16, 2010) (*National Broadband Plan*).

[11] As defined in the *National Broadband Plan,* Health IT includes "information-driven health practices and the technologies that enable them" such as "billing and scheduling systems, e-care, EHRs, telehealth and mobile health." *Id.*

[12] Telehealth is defined as the "electronic exchange of information–data, images and video–to aid in the practice of medicine, advanced analytics" and non-clinical practices such as continuing medical education and nursing call centers. It encompasses technologies that enable video consultation, remote monitoring and image transmission (store-and-forward) over fixed or mobile networks. *Id.*

[13] Although related to telehealth, telemedicine is usually more narrowly defined. The Centers for Medicare and Medicaid Services (CMS) defines "telemedicine" as "two-way, real time interactive communication between the patient, and the physician or practitioner at the distant site to improve a patient's health." Centers for Medicare & Medicaid Services, http://www.medicaid.gov/Medicaid-CHIP-Program-Information/By-Topics/Delivery-Systems/Telemedicine.html (last visited Apr. 19, 2012). The American Telemedicine Association defines "telemedicine" as "the use of medical information exchanged from one site to another via electronic communications to improve patients' health status." American Telemedicine Association, http://www.americantelemed.org/i4a/pages/index.cfm?pageid=3333 (last visited June 5, 2012).

[14] The *National Broadband Plan* defines an EHR as "a digital record of patient health information generated by one or more encounters in any care delivery setting." It includes "patient demographics, progress notes, diagnoses,

(continued . . .)

increased rural health care providers' need for robust broadband connections. Since the *2006 Pilot Program Order*, rural health care providers have continued to use telemedicine to improve and reduce the cost of health care for their patients. For people living in rural areas, travel time to locations where specialists practice can be substantial, and the associated delay in obtaining treatment can have serious consequences. There are shortages of physicians in many rural areas, and Pilot projects have used their networks to meet the health care needs of their patients and accomplish other telehealth purposes.[15] In addition, there have been significant advances in the move to adoption and exchange of electronic health records. Most notably, in the 2009 HITECH Act, Congress adopted an incentive payment system under Medicare and Medicaid to encourage health care providers to convert to electronic health records and to develop the capability of exchanging those records.[16] Since that time, a number of health care providers have been working towards the adoption and exchange of electronic health records.

7. Many Pilot projects have made substantial advances towards completion. About half of the total Pilot funding had been committed as of January 2012, and USAC estimates that by the end of 2012, total funding requested and processed will be approximately $368 million (a figure equal to 95 percent of the 50 active projects' cumulative total original awards). Furthermore, about a quarter of individual health care provider sites will have spent their allotment of Pilot Program funds by June 30, 2013.[17] Given the extent of the Commission's experience to date with the Pilot Program, coupled with recent developments in Health IT, the time is ripe to evaluate the Pilot Program so that the Commission may draw on that experience in considering reforms to the RHC program in the pending rulemaking proceeding.[18] Accordingly, the Bureau staff has prepared this Report, which is divided into four parts: (1) the creation and design of the Pilot Program; (2) the description of the Pilot projects and their network characteristics; (3) the improved quality and reduced cost of health care realized by the projects as a result of their broadband networks; and (4) key observations regarding the Pilot Program.

II. BACKGROUND

A. The Creation of the Rural Health Care Support Mechanism

8. As part of the Telecommunications Act of 1996 (1996 Act), Congress directed the Commission to provide rural health care providers with "an affordable rate for the services necessary for

---

(. . . continued from previous page) ─────────────────────────────

medications, vital signs, medical history, immunizations, laboratory data and radiology reports." *National Broadband Plan* at 200.

[15] *See* USAC Mar. 16 Site Visit Reports at 6, 14 (observing that Henry County Health Center, a rural health care provider participating in the Iowa Rural Health Telecommunication Program, and rural health care providers in the Avera Health network respectively use tele-radiology and tele-pharmacy to meet the health care needs of their patients). *See also* NARMH Apr. 12 *Ex Parte* Letter at 1 (explaining that telemedicine allows patients to be cared for in their communities even when a physician is not physically located at that site); ONC Jan. 17 *Ex Parte* Letter at 2 (the "shortage of physicians in rural areas means that there is even more need to leverage technology and use telehealth to provide care to patients in rural areas"); Pilot Project Conference Call Mar. 13 *Ex Parte* Letter (PMHA *et al.*) at 1 (noting that South Carolina faces challenges to similar to most rural states, including a paucity of specialized services).

[16] *See* Letter from Kathleen Sebelius, Secretary of Health and Human Services, to Julius Genachowski, Chairman, FCC, WC Docket No. 02-60 (filed Sept. 7, 2010) at 1 (HHS Comments).

[17] USAC Aug. 2 Data Letter at 2.

[18] *See 2010 NPRM; see also 2006 Pilot Program Order,* 21 FCC Rcd at 11112, para. 4.

the provision of telemedicine and instruction relating to such services."[19] Specifically, the 1996 Act mandated that telecommunications carriers provide telecommunications services for health care purposes to rural public or non-profit health care providers at rates that were "reasonably comparable" to rates in urban areas.[20] However, not all public or non-profit health care providers are eligible to participate. Eligible health care providers, as defined in the 1996 Act, only include (1) post-secondary educational institutions offering health care instruction, teaching hospitals, and medical schools; (2) community health centers or health centers providing health care to migrants; (3) local health departments or agencies; (4) community mental health centers; (5) not-for-profit hospitals; (6) rural health clinics; and (7) consortia of health care providers consisting of one or more entities falling into the first six categories.[21]

9.   Consistent with Congress's directive, the Commission established the rural health care telecommunications program in 1997 to ensure that rural health care providers pay no more than their urban counterparts for their telecommunications needs in the provision of health care services.[22] The telecommunications program ensures that eligible rural health care providers can obtain a rate for each supported service that is no higher than the highest tariffed or publicly available commercial rate for a similar service in the closest city in the state with a population of 50,000 or more people, taking distance charges into account – in effect, providing a discount to the HCP in the amount of the "rural-urban differential."[23]

10. In 2003, the Commission created the rural health care Internet access program pursuant to section 254(h)(2)(A) of the Act, which directs the Commission to establish competitively neutral rules to enhance, to the extent technically feasible and economically reasonable, access to "advanced telecommunications and information services" for public and non-profit health care providers.[24] The Internet access program provides a 25 percent discount off the cost of monthly Internet access for eligible rural health care providers.[25] Together the telecommunications and Internet access programs are commonly referred to as the "Primary Program."

---

[19] Telecommunications Act of 1996, Pub. L. No. 104-104, 110 Stat. 56 (1996). The 1996 Act amended the Communications Act of 1934 (Communications Act or Act); Joint Explanatory Statement of the Committee of Conference, 104th Cong., 2d Sess. at 133 (1996); *see also* 47 U.S.C. § 254(b)(3), (h).

[20] *See* 47 U.S.C. § 254(h)(1)(A) (directing that telecommunications carriers should provide "telecommunications services" that are necessary for the provision of health care services to any "public or nonprofit" health care provider that serves persons who reside in rural areas, at rates that are "reasonably comparable" to rates in urban areas).

[21] 47 U.S.C. § 254(h)(7)(B).

[22] *See, e.g.*, 47 U.S.C. § 254(h)(1)(A); *Federal-State Joint Board on Universal Service*, CC Docket No. 96-45, Report and Order, 12 FCC Rcd 8776, 9093-9161, paras. 608-749 (1997) (*Universal Service First Report and Order*) (subsequent history omitted); 47 C.F.R. Part 54, Subpart G.

[23] *Universal Service First Report and Order,* 12 FCC Rcd at 9093, para. 608.

[24] 47 U.S.C. § 254(h)(2)(A).

[25] 47 C.F.R. § 54.621. *See generally Rural Health Care Support Mechanism*, WC Docket No. 02-60, Report and Order, Order on Reconsideration, and Further Notice of Proposed Rulemaking, 18 FCC Rcd 24546 (2003) (*2003 Order and Further Notice*). A 50 percent discount (rather than 25 percent) is available for Internet access services for health care providers in states that are "entirely rural," that is, states in which every county meets the Commission's definition of rural. *Rural Health Care Support Mechanism*, WC Docket No. 02-60, Second Report and Order, Order on Reconsideration, and Further Notice of Proposed Rulemaking, 19 FCC Rcd 24613, 24631, para. 38 (2004) (*Second Report and Order and Further Notice*).

11. As of June 30, 2011, approximately $414 million had been disbursed through the Primary Program.[26] Annual disbursements have grown through the course of the Primary Program, from $3.375 million in 1998 (the first funding year), to $10 million in 2000, $25 million in 2003, $54 million in 2007, and $81.5 million in 2010.[27]

B. The Creation of the Pilot Program

12. In September 2006, the Commission established the Rural Health Care Pilot Program to provide funding to support state or regional broadband networks designed to bring the benefits of innovative telehealth and telemedicine services to those areas of the country where the need for those benefits is most acute.[28] The Pilot Program provides funding for up to 85 percent of the costs associated with: (1) the construction of state or regional broadband networks, and the advanced telecommunications and information services provided over those networks; (2) connecting to nationwide backbone providers Internet2 or National LambdaRail (NLR); and (3) connecting to the public Internet.[29] Pilot projects can use RHC support to purchase services from third parties, or to receive service by constructing and owning their own network facilities.[30] Additionally, the Pilot Program allows participants to use funding to purchase items that are not eligible for support under the Primary Program, such as equipment (*e.g.* servers, routers, firewalls, switches, and other devices or equipment necessary for the broadband connection), or to upgrade their existing equipment and increase bandwidth.[31]

13. In creating the Pilot Program, the Commission noted that broadband was enabling health care providers to vastly improve access to quality medical services in remote areas of the country, but that health care providers lacked access to the broadband facilities needed to support the types of advanced telehealth applications, such as telemedicine, that are so vital to bringing medical expertise and the advantages of modern health care technology to rural areas of the country.[32] The Commission stated that even though it had taken a number of steps to spur deployment of the type of broadband facilities that would support advanced medical technologies, the RHC support mechanism had to date not adequately provided the type of support needed to encourage development of dedicated broadband

---

[26] *See* Universal Service Monitoring Report, Dec. 2011, CC Docket No. 98-202, Table 2.21, *available at* http://www fcc.gov/wcb/stats (last visited May 7, 2012) (*2011 Universal Service Monitoring Report*).

[27] *See id.*; Universal Service Administrative Company, 2011 Annual Report at 13, *available at* http://www.usac.org/about/tools/publications/annual-reports/2011/index html (last visited Apr. 17, 2012) (2011 USAC Annual Report).

[28] *2006 Pilot Program Order,* 21 FCC Rcd at 11111, para. 1.

[29] *2007 Pilot Program Selection Order*, 22 FCC Rcd at 20361, para. 2.

[30] *See 2006 Pilot Program Order*, 21 FCC Rcd at 11111, para. 1, 11115-16, paras. 14-15. In the *2007 Pilot Program Selection Order*, the Commission clarified that, to the extent a selected participant leases transmission services in lieu of deploying its own broadband network, the costs for subscribing to such facilities and services are eligible for program support. *2007 Pilot Program Selection Order*, 22 FCC Rcd at 20397-98, para. 74. Throughout this Report, we distinguish between services purchased by HCPs from third parties (which may include mechanisms such as long-term leases, prepaid leases, and indefeasible rights of use of facilities for specified period of time (IRUs)) from "self-construction" (*i.e.* network facilities constructed and owned by the HCPs).

[31] *2007 Pilot Program Selection Order*, 22 FCC Rcd at 20397-98, para. 74. *See also* USAC Observations Letter at 6-7 (explaining that unlike Primary Program participants, Pilot Program participants could use RHC support to purchase and upgrade their equipment if necessary).

[32] *2006 Pilot Program Order,* 21 FCC Rcd at 11113, para. 8.

networks among health care providers.[33] The Pilot Program was intended to "provide the Commission with a more complete and practical understanding of how to ensure the best use of the available RHC support mechanism funds to support a broadband, nationwide health care network (expressly including rural areas) so that the Commission can reform the overall RHC support mechanism."[34]

14. *Selection of Pilot Projects.* Given the nature of the Pilot Program, the Commission encouraged multiple health care providers in a state or region to join together to formulate and submit proposals.[35] Pilot Program applicants were instructed to present a strategy for aggregating the specific needs of health care providers within a state or region, including providers that serve rural areas, and for leveraging existing technology to adopt the most efficient and cost-effective means of connecting those providers.[36] While participation was opened to all eligible public and non-profit health care providers, applicants were required to include in their proposed networks more than a *de minimis* number of health care providers that serve rural areas.[37] The *2006 Pilot Program Order* also included 11 specific criteria that applicants were instructed to address in their applications, including the proposed network's goals and objectives, previous experience in developing and managing telemedicine programs, and the extent to which the network would be self-sustaining once established.[38]

---

[33] *Id.* While the Primary Program provides rural health care providers with substantial telecommunications and Internet discounts, in its *2006 Pilot Program Order*, the Commission recognized that the program had yet to fully achieve the benefits intended by the statute and the Commission. Although the Primary Program was capped at $400 million, since the program's inception in 1998 through 2006, the program generally had disbursed less than 10 percent of the cap each year. *Id.*

[34] *Id.* at 11113, para. 9; *see also 2007 Pilot Program Selection Order*, 22 FCC Rcd at 20366-67, para. 15.

[35] *2006 Pilot Program Order*, 21 FCC Rcd at 11111, para. 3.

[36] *Id.* at 11116, para. 16.

[37] *Id.* at 11111, 11114, paras. 3, 10. The Pilot Program was established under section 254(h)(2)(A) of the Act, which provides the Commission broad discretionary authority to provide universal service support for "advanced services" for all health care providers. See 47 U.S.C. § 254(h)(2)(A) ("the Commission shall establish competitively neutral rules to enhance, to the extent technically feasible and economically reasonable, access to advanced telecommunications and information services for all public and nonprofit ... health care providers"); *Texas Office of Public Utility Counsel v. FCC*, 18 F.3d 393, 446 (5th Cir. 1999) (concluding that "the language in § 254(h)(2)(A) demonstrates Congress's intent to authorize expanding support to 'advanced services,' when possible, for non-rural health providers").

[38] *2006 Pilot Program Order*, 21 FCC Rcd at 11116-17, para. 17. The remaining applicant criteria included the following: (1) identify the organization that will be legally and financially responsible for the conduct of activities supported by the fund; (2) estimate the network's total costs for each year; (3) describe how for-profit network participants will pay their fair share of the network costs; (4) identify the source of financial support and anticipated revenues that will pay for costs not covered by the fund; (5) list the health care facilities that will be included in the network; (6) provide the address, zip code, Rural Urban Commuting Area (RUCA) code, and phone number for each health care facility participating in the network; (7) provide a project management plan outlining the project's leadership and management structure, as well as its work plan, schedule, and budget; and (8) indicate how the telemedicine program will be coordinated throughout the state or region. *Id.* In addition, applicants were instructed to demonstrate that they have a viable strategic plan for aggregating usage among health care providers within their state or region. *Id.* at 11116, para. 16. In selecting participants for the Pilot Program, the Commission also indicated that it would consider whether an applicant has had a successful track record in developing, coordinating, and implementing a successful telehealth/telemedicine program within their state or region, and the number of health care providers that are included in the proposed network, with considerable weight given to applications that propose to connect the rural health care providers in a given state or region. *Id.*

15. The Pilot Program generated overwhelming interest from the health care community, and the Commission received 81 applications representing approximately 6,800 health care providers.[39] On November 16, 2007, the Commission selected 69 Pilot Program applications covering 42 states and three United States territories.[40] The Commission awarded these 69 projects approximately $418 million in total to construct or lease state or local regional broadband networks and provide advanced communications services over their networks.[41] Individual project awards, which were initially to be utilized over a three-year period, ranged from about $93,000 to almost $25 million.[42]

16. The 69 selected applicants demonstrated to the Commission their overall qualifications, consistent with the goals of the Pilot Program, to stimulate deployment of the broadband infrastructure necessary to support innovative telehealth and, in particular, telemedicine services to those areas of the country where the need for those benefits is most acute.[43] The Commission explained that the selected participants, among other things, described strategies for aggregating the specific needs of health care providers within a state or region, including providers serving rural areas; provided strategies for leveraging existing technology to adopt the most efficient and cost-effective means of connecting those providers; described previous experience in developing and managing telemedicine programs; and had detailed project management plans.[44] Rather than limiting participation to a select few among the 69 qualified applicants, the Commission found that it would be in the best interests of the Pilot Program, and appropriate as a matter of universal service policy, to accommodate as many of the qualified applicants as possible.[45]

C. Application Process

17. Selected Pilot Program participants are required to follow the normal Primary Program procedures, as modified for the Pilot Program.[46] The steps required for Pilot participants include the following:

- **Organize Project and Prepare for Competitive Bidding:** Each Pilot project must identify a lead entity and project coordinators, obtain letters of agency from each

---

[39] *2007 Pilot Program Selection Order*, 22 FCC Rcd at 20370, para. 22; *see also Wireline Competition Bureau Announces OMB Approval of the Rural Health Care Pilot Program Information Collection Requirements and the Deadline for Filing Applications*, WC Docket No. 02-60, Public Notice, 22 FCC Rcd 4770 (Wireline Comp. Bur. 2007).

[40] *2007 Pilot Program Selection Order*, 22 FCC Rcd at 20370, para. 22.

[41] *See id.* at 20360, 20429-30, App. B. As a result of the merger of certain projects, the withdrawal of others, and the failure of some to meet certain deadlines, there are currently 50 active projects in the Pilot Program. *See infra* Section III.A.

[42] *2007 Pilot Program Selection Order*, 22 FCC Rcd at 20361, para 2. The lowest award was for $93,240 (Mountain States Health Care Alliance); the highest was $24,689,016 (New England Telehealth Consortium). *See* Fig. 2, below; USAC May 4 Data Letter at 2.

[43] *Id.* at 20370, para. 22.

[44] *Id.*

[45] *2007 Pilot Program Selection Order*, 22 FCC Rcd at 20370, para. 22.

[46] *See 2006 Pilot Program Order*, 21 FCC Rcd at 11115, para. 13 & n.19; *see also 2007 Pilot Program Selection Order*, 22 FCC Rcd at 20403-04, para. 83.

participating health care provider, determine network configuration, identify source for 15 percent match, and prepare a Request for Proposal (RFP).[47]

- **Post Request for Services (Form 465)**: Each Pilot project must file Form 465 (which includes an RFP and other required documentation) and obtain USAC verification of eligibility of participating HCPs; USAC posts Form 465 on its web site, which starts the competitive bidding process.[48]

- **Select Vendor and Contract for Services:** Each Pilot project must review bids, select a vendor, and negotiate and execute a contract. Projects must wait at least 28 days after posting of the RFP before committing to a particular vendor.[49]

- **Obtain USAC Funding "Commitment" (Form 466-A)**: Each Pilot project must file the required documentation notifying USAC of the vendor selected and the associated cost (Form 466-A).[50] After reviewing, USAC "commits" the funds (*i.e.*, will issue a "Funding Commitment Letter" (FCL) specifying the amount of support).[51]

- **Receive Services and Notify USAC (Form 467):** The Pilot project orders the service from the vendor, receives services, and notifies USAC that services have been initiated. The vendor can then send the invoices to the project, which the project reviews and forwards to USAC. USAC will then "disburse" the funds to the vendor. Projects have six years from issuance of the initial funding commitment letter to invoice USAC.[52]

18. In addition to complying with the modified Primary Program procedures detailed above, Pilot Program participants must submit to the Commission and USAC quarterly reports detailing, among other things, project management, included health care facilities, network specifications, costs, and advancement of telemedicine benefits.[53] Participants must state in these quarterly reports whether their networks are or will become self-sustaining and, if so, how their networks are self-sustaining.[54]

D.   Post-Selection Developments

19. Since 2007, the Pilot Program has gone through many changes. Although the Pilot Program was intended to be a three-year program with funding evenly allocated in Funding Years 2007-09, it has taken more time than originally anticipated for the projects to identify their needs, design their networks,

---

[47] *2007 Pilot Program Selection Order*, 22 FCC Rcd at 20403-06, paras. 83, 85-87.

[48] *Id.* at 20412, para. 100.

[49] *See* 47 C.F.R. § 54.603(b)(3).

[50] *2007 Pilot Program Selection Order*, 22 FCC Rcd at 20403, para. 83.

[51] *Id.* at 20409, para 93. Pursuant to the Commission's rules, a rural health care funding year runs from July 1 through June 30 and rural health care support recipients, including Pilot Program participants, must submit their FCC Forms 466-A for a given funding year by the end of that funding year, *i.e.*, by June 30. *See* 47 C.F.R. § 54.623(b)-(c); *see also* FCC Form 466-A Instructions, *available at* http://www.usac.org/rhc/tools/required-forms.aspx.

[52] *Rural Health Care Support Mechanism,* WC Docket No. 02-60, Order, 26 FCC Rcd 6619, 6628, para. 19 (Wireline Comp. Bur. 2011) (*2011 Extension Order*). For instance, if a particular participant received its initial funding commitment on April 7, 2011, it is required to complete invoicing by April 7, 2017.

[53] *2007 Pilot Program Selection Order*, 22 FCC Rcd at 20423-24, para. 126, App. D.

[54] *Id.* at 20416, para. 108, App. D.

secure funding for administrative expenses, complete the application process, prepare RFPs, conduct competitive bidding, and enter into contracts with vendors. In response, the Bureau has extended the program to accommodate the projects' needs. First, the Bureau permitted projects to carry over unused funds from year to year during the duration of the award.[55] Second, the Bureau extended the time for projects to receive funding commitments from USAC for the entirety of their awards from June 30, 2010 to June 30, 2012.[56] Finally, the Bureau extended the deadline for projects to invoice USAC for disbursements from five years to six.[57] As a result, Pilot projects have had more time than originally provided in the *2007 Pilot Program Selection Order* to create their networks.

20. *Project Mergers and Withdrawals.* Of the original 69 projects, several have merged, withdrawn from the program, or failed to meet program deadlines, leaving the total number of projects currently in the Pilot Program at 50. Appendix A lists the status of the 69 original awardees, by lead state.

- *Mergers:* From 2008 to 2009, projects merged in Mississippi, North Carolina, Ohio, Pennsylvania and Texas, leaving a total of 62 projects.[58]

- *Withdrawals:* An additional four of the 62 remaining projects withdrew from the Pilot Program due to financial constraints, competitive bidding issues, or lack of health care provider (HCP) interest. The awards to these four projects accounted for about $4.7 million, or about 1 percent, of the Pilot Program.[59]

- *Failed to Meet Program Deadlines:* In May 2011, the Bureau issued an order granting one-year extensions of program deadlines for Pilot Program participants, subject to the condition that the participant must have chosen a vendor and filed at least one complete request for funding before June 30, 2011.[60] The Bureau stated that projects that failed to meet the June 30, 2011, deadline for filing at least one complete request for funding would be deemed "no longer capable of continuing in the Pilot Program," and would "not be given additional time beyond that date to request Pilot Program funding."[61] Of the remaining 58 projects, eight projects did not meet the June 30, 2011 deadline.[62] Two projects were able to accomplish their goals with alternate funding sources.[63] One project intended to use Pilot funds for ineligible costs (personnel) and could not restructure its proposal in a way that attracted HCP interest. Five projects, for other reasons, did not proceed with their projects on a timely

---

[55] Letter from Dana R. Shaffer, Chief, Wireline Competition Bureau, to Scott Barash, Acting Chief Executive Officer, Universal Service Administrative Company (Jan. 17, 2008), *available at* http://hraunfoss fcc.gov/edocs_public/attachmatch/DOC-279603A1.pdf.

[56] *See Rural Health Care Support Mechanism,* WC Docket No. 02-60, Order, 25 FCC Rcd 1423 (Wireline Comp. Bur. 2010) (*2010 Extension Order*); *see also 2011 Extension Order*, 26 FCC Rcd 6619.

[57] *2011 Extension Order,* 26 FCC Rcd at 6628, para. 19.

[58] A total of 12 projects merged in these five states. *See* USAC May 4 Data Letter at 1-2.

[59] USAC May 4 Data Letter at 2. The four projects were the Alabama Pediatric Health Access Network, Rural Healthcare Association of Alabama, KanEd, and the Healthcare Education and Research Network.

[60] *2011 Extension Order*, 26 FCC Rcd at 6625, para. 10.

[61] *Id.* at 6625, 6628, paras. 10, 22.

[62] USAC May 4 Data Letter at 2.

[63] *Id.*

basis.[64] These eight projects accounted for about $25.1 million, or about 6 percent of the Pilot Program.[65]

21. In July 2010, the Commission issued a notice of proposed rulemaking seeking comment on several proposed reforms to the RHC support mechanism.[66] The reforms included a proposal to create a new health infrastructure program that would support up to 85 percent of the construction costs of new regional or statewide networks to serve public and non-profit health care providers in areas of the country where broadband is insufficient or unavailable.[67] Additionally, the *2010 NPRM* also included a proposal to establish a health broadband services program that would support up to 50 percent of the monthly recurring costs for access to broadband services for eligible public or non-profit health care providers.[68] The *2010 NPRM* is currently pending. In November 2010, the Government Accountability Office recommended, in part, that the Commission develop and execute a sound performance evaluation plan for the current programs, and develop sound evaluation plans as part of the design of any new programs proposed in the *2010 NPRM*.[69]

22. In an order released July 6, 2012, the Commission provided temporary "bridge" funding to those Pilot projects with sites that will have exhausted their Pilot funding before the end of funding year 2013 (before June 30, 2013), in order to maintain the status quo for these projects while a process is established to transition them into a permanent rural health care support mechanism.[70] In a Public Notice released July 19, 2012, the Wireline Competition Bureau sought additional comment on several issues in the *2010 NPRM*, in order to develop a more robust record, particularly in light of the experience in the Pilot Program since the issuance of the *NPRM*.[71]

III.   DESCRIPTION OF THE PILOT PROJECTS

23. In this section we describe the characteristics of the Pilot projects. Each project is by definition a consortium of individual health care providers. We first detail the varying size of the projects in terms of the number of health care providers participating in each project. We then describe the funding awards, commitments, and disbursements for the projects.[72] Of the 69 that received funding awards under the Pilot Program, 50 projects are currently active and have received funding commitments. As detailed above, the 19 projects that are no longer active either have merged with other projects or, for a variety of reasons, have withdrawn or have been disqualified from participating in the Program.[73]

---

[64] *Id.*

[65] *Id.*

[66] *See 2010 NPRM*, 25 FCC Rcd 9371.

[67] *Id.* at 9373, para. 3.

[68] *Id.*

[69] *GAO Report* at 56-57.

[70] *Rural Health Care Support Mechanism,* Order, WC Docket No. 02-60, FCC 12-74 (rel. July 6, 2012) (*Bridge Funding Order*).

[71] *Rural Health Care Support Mechanism,* WC Docket No. 02-60, Public Notice, DA 12-1166 (Wireline Comp. Bureau, rel. July 19, 2012).

[72] *See supra* Section II.C. for an explanation of "commitments" and "disbursements."

[73] *See supra* Section II.D.

24. We then detail the geographic coverage of the active Pilot projects, which include sites in 38 states and three territories. Most projects include urban health care providers but most projects are predominantly made up of rural health care providers.[74] This section also details the number and type of health care providers participating in the projects, as well as their network design and architecture.

25. Finally, we describe how the networks have been implemented and the types of broadband services utilized by the projects. Many of the projects chose to purchase broadband services from third parties rather than construct and operate a broadband network themselves. As intended, most health care providers participating in the Pilot Program obtained the high-bandwidth broadband connections sufficient to support health IT applications. The Pilot Program also has enabled many of the projects to exercise increased purchasing power and secure more advantageous pricing than would generally have been possible for an individual health care provider.

A.   Size of Projects and Awards

26. *Size of Projects.* Pilot projects vary widely in size depending on their scope. For example, Palmetto State Providers Network (PSPN), a statewide backbone network that connects rural and underserved areas in South Carolina, includes 120 to 150 health care provider sites in all 46 counties of the state.[75] On the other hand, Pennsylvania Mountains Healthcare Alliance (PMHA), a regional network located in central and western Pennsylvania, is comprised of only 21 hospitals.[76] In their original proposals, Pilot projects identified over 6,400 health care providers that expressed interest in participating in their networks.[77] As of the end of January 2012, USAC had verified the eligibility of 5,475 health care providers participating in Pilot Program networks and issued funding commitments to approximately 2,100 health care providers.[78]

27. Twelve projects had ten or fewer sites in their original proposals. At the other end of the spectrum, 18 projects had over 100 sites in their original proposals.[79] The projects still range widely in size, as shown in Figure 1. As of January 2012, about a third of active projects included at least 50 individual health care providers that had received funding commitments. Another third had 11 to 50 such providers. Of the remaining third, some projects are lagging behind in implementation, but several are smaller projects (fewer than 10 health care providers) by design. Seven of the projects had received funding commitments for only one site as of January 2012.[80] As noted above, USAC has received many funding commitment requests since January 31, 2012, and the deadline for filing all funding commitment requests was June 30, 2012. When those requests are all processed, the numbers of HCPs in many of the projects will likely be higher.

---

[74] Due to the inherent limitations of the Commission's definition of "rural" (or any definition of "rural"), the term "urban" can include sites located in relatively sparsely-populated areas. For example, Orangeburg County Clinic in Holly Hill, SC (pop. 1,277), a health care provider participating in Palmetto State Providers Network's Pilot project, is characterized as "urban." The largest cities closest to Holly Hill are Charleston, SC, and Columbia, SC, respectively 50 and 69 miles away from Holly Hill.

[75] Pilot Conference Call Mar. 13 *Ex Parte* Letter (PMHA *et al.*) at 1.

[76] *Id.*

[77] USAC May 4 Data Letter at 1.

[78] USAC 2011 Annual Report at 12.

[79] *See* Fig. 1.

[80] The seven projects that have received only one funding commitment letter to date have proposed to include multiple sites as required by the *2006 Pilot Program Order*, but had not yet received funding commitments for those additional sites as of January 2012.

Figure 1 – Project Size (By Number of HCPs)[81]

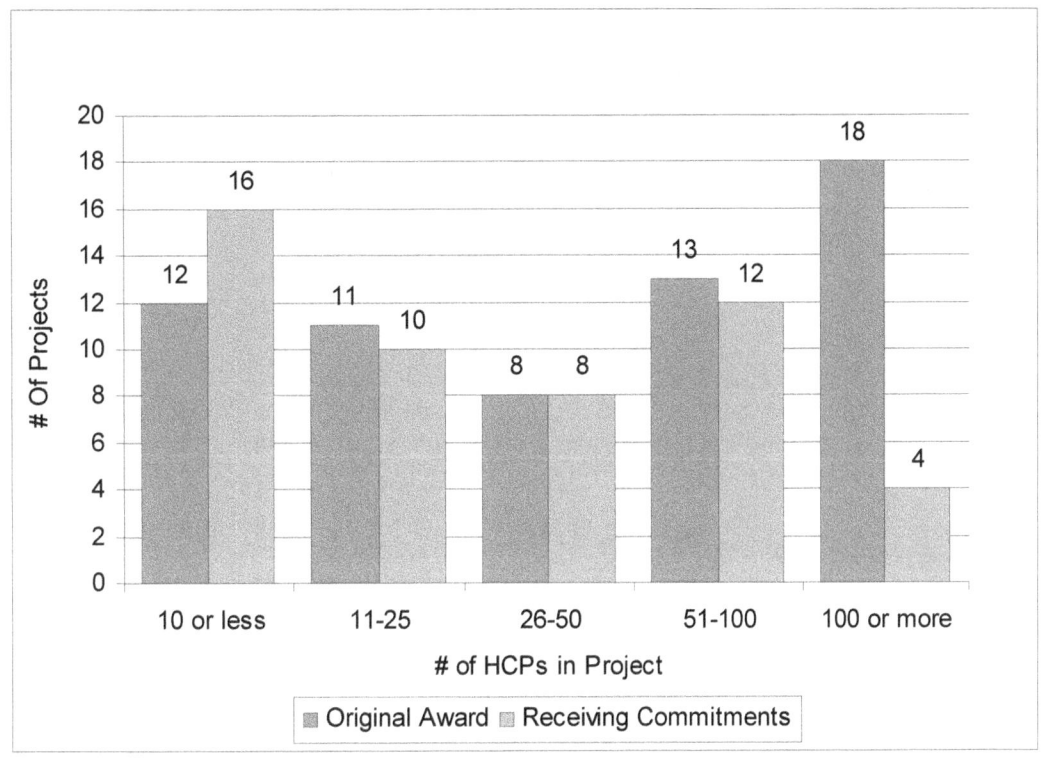

28. *Awards, Commitments, and Disbursements.* Figure 2 shows the award for each of the original 69 pilot projects, from low to high. Total project awards ranged from $93,240 to $24,689,016.[82] Support per site ranged from $3,400 to as much as $2.5 million, with an average of $70,000 per site.[83]

---

[81] USAC Data Letter Aug. 9 at App. D. All projects proposed, and intend, to connect multiple health care providers. As of January 31, 2012, there were seven projects with only one HCP receiving a funding commitment. Four of these projects were instructed by USAC to assign the cost of the network design study to the lead entity (consortium), resulting in the data showing only one HCP receiving a commitment for those projects that had not yet implemented their networks as of January 31, 2012. The remaining three projects filed a commitment request for only one HCP in order to meet the June 30, 2011 deadline to request at least one commitment. *See id.*

[82] *2007 Pilot Program Selection Order*, 22 FCC Rcd at 20429-30, App. B.

[83] USAC Observations Letter at 1.

Figure 2 – Pilot Projects – Original Award Amount[84]

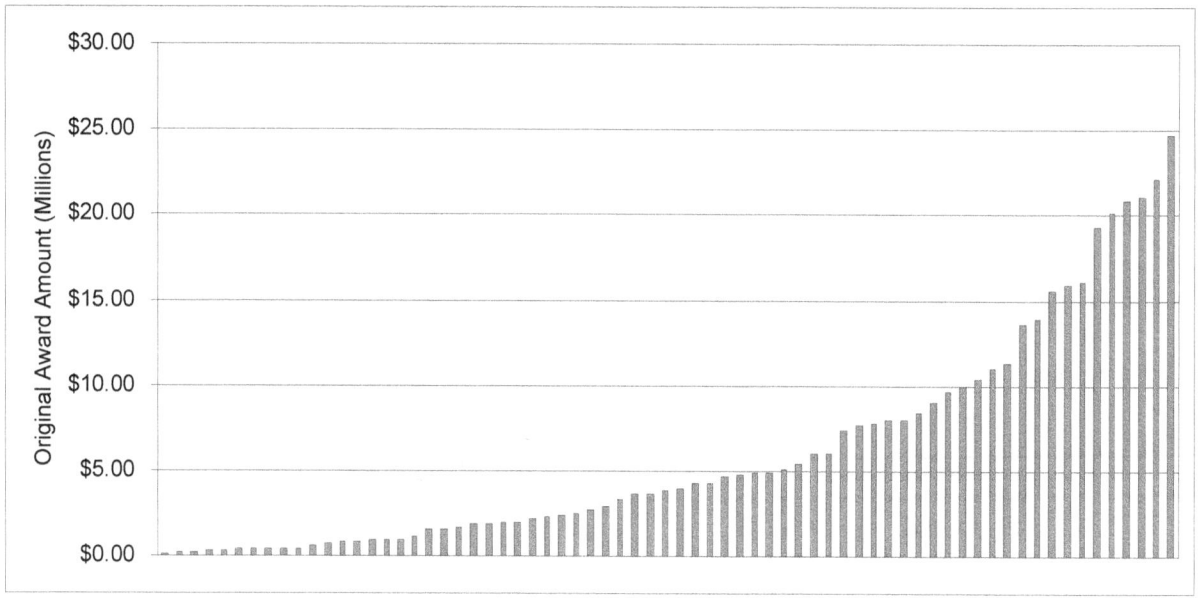

29. One way to measure the progress of projects is to review what percentage of the original award has been *committed* (*i.e.,* the project can begin receiving services because it has completed competitive bidding, selected a vendor, and signed a contract) and *disbursed* (*i.e.,* the project has received services and the vendor has been reimbursed by USAC). Figures 3(a) and 3(b) show the Pilot projects by the percentages of awards that have been committed and disbursed, respectively, as of January 30, 2012. The percentage of each project's award that has been committed and disbursed varies significantly across projects.

---

[84] *2007 Pilot Program Selection Order*, 22 FCC Rcd at 20429-30, App. B.

Figure 3(a) – Pilot Projects, Percentage of Award Committed[85]

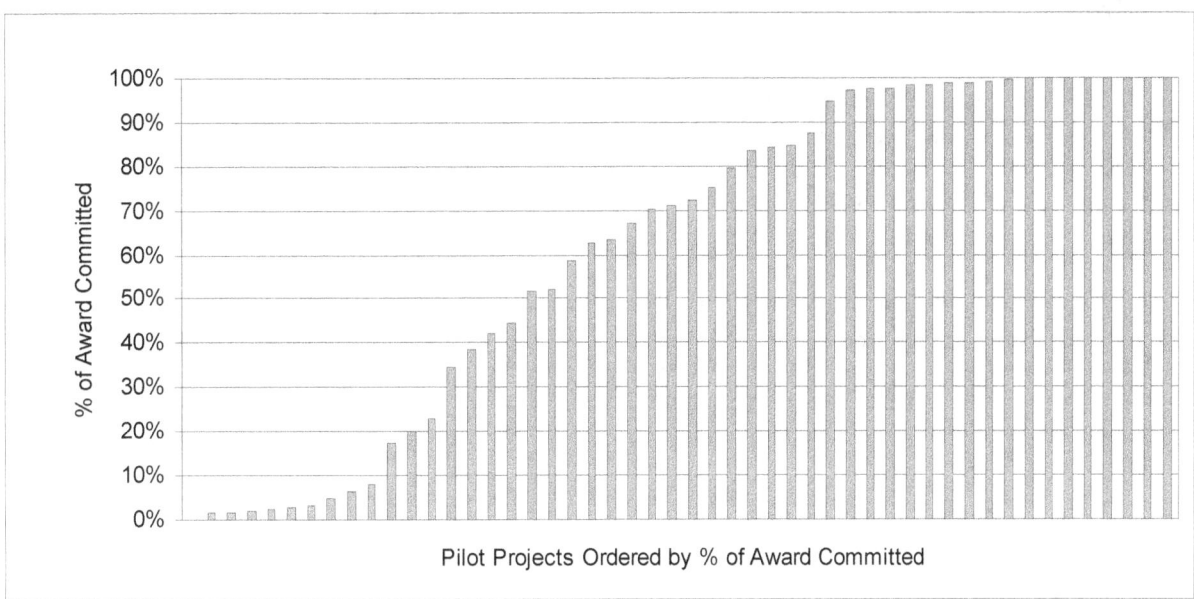

Figure 3(b) – Pilot Projects, Percentage of Award Disbursed[86]

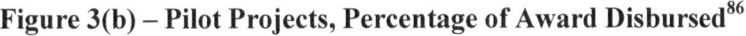

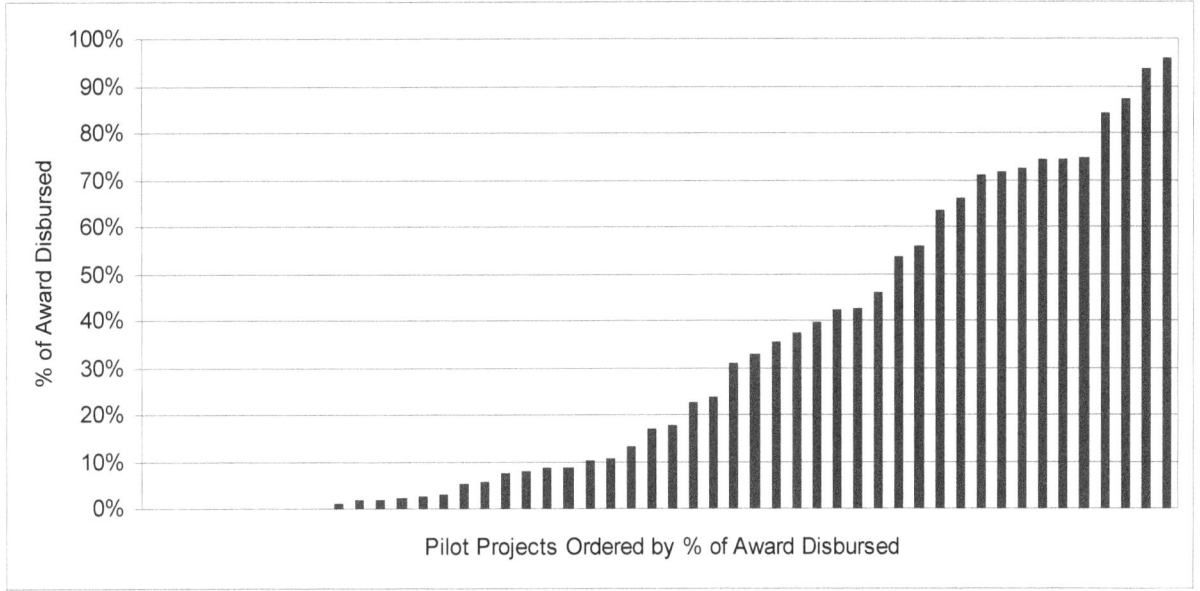

30. *Commitments.* As of the end of January 2012, USAC had committed $217 million to approximately 2,100 health care providers participating in the Pilot Program, or about $100,000 on average per health care provider.[87] About two-thirds of active Pilot projects had received commitments

---

[85] USAC Data Letter Aug. 9 at App. A.

[86] *Id.* at App. B.

[87] USAC Data Letter May 4 at 2. By way of comparison, from January 1, 1998 through January 31, 2012, the Primary Program had committed $232 million to 5,536 health care providers (excluding Alaska) (or about $45,000 each), with an additional $273 million committed to 283 Alaska health care providers. *Id.* at 2-3. Health care providers in Alaska face unique costs because the state's vast size, harsh winter weather, and sparse population

(continued . . .)

for the majority of their individual awards, while 44 percent of projects had received commitments for 81 percent or more of their awards.[88] On the other hand, about a quarter of projects had yet to obtain commitments for more than 20 percent of their awards by this date.[89]

31. The deadline for submitting all remaining requests for funding was June 30, 2012.[90] As of July 3, 2012, USAC had received requests from all 50 active projects and had 108 funding requests to be processed.[91] The 108 pending funding requests represent approximately $91.60 million for 30 projects; USAC estimates that once processed, total funding commitments requested will be $368.62 million, which is 88.23 percent of the original total award amount of $417.78 million.[92]

32. *Disbursements.* As of the end of January 2012, USAC had disbursed approximately $100 million, or half of the amount for which Pilot projects had received funding commitments.[93] Because each project has up to six years from issuance of its first funding commitment letter to complete its invoicing, the rate of disbursements lags behind the rate of commitments.[94] While slow initially, disbursement amounts have accelerated each year of the Pilot Program, as shown in Figure 4 below.

33. Figure 3(b) above shows that projects are in widely different stages of completion and spending. Only about 28 percent of projects (14) had received disbursements of over half of their award, as of January 30, 2012.[95] About a quarter of the projects had received disbursements of less than 20 percent of their awards by that date.[96] On the other hand, some advanced projects have HCPs nearing the conclusion of Pilot-funded activity within the next funding year.[97] USAC estimates that during the 2012 funding year (July 2012 to June 2013), approximately 484 HCPs in 14 projects, or approximately a quarter of HCPs participating in the Pilot Program, will have spent all of the Pilot money allocated within the project's Pilot award.[98] As noted above, in an order released July 6, 2012, the Commission

(. . . continued from previous page) ————————————————

make it challenging to deploy fiber or wireless networks in many rural areas. In many parts of rural Alaska, expensive satellite services may be the only option available.

[88] USAC Aug. 2 Data Letter at 2. In some cases, Pilot projects may not seek commitments for the full amount of their awards – if, for example, the competitive bidding process or other cost savings allow the project to achieve its goals for less than the amount requested in the project's initial application.

[89] *Id.*

[90] The original deadline for requesting all remaining funding for the Pilot Program on FCC Form 466-A was June 30, 2010. *2007 Pilot Program Selection Order*, 22 FCC Rcd at 20370, para. 23. The Bureau has twice extended the deadline for submitting requests for funding. June 30, 2011 was the deadline for projects to receive their first funding commitment letter or file a complete Form 466-A packet with USAC. *2011 Extension Order*, 26 FCC Rcd at 6626-27, para. 14. June 30, 2012 is the deadline for projects to request all remaining funding in their award on FCC Form 466-A. *Id.* at 6627-8, para. 18.

[91] USAC Aug. 2 Data Letter at 2.

[92] *Id.*

[93] USAC May 4 Data Letter at 3.

[94] *2007 Pilot Program Selection Order*, 22 FCC Rcd at 20370, para. 94. *See also supra Section* II.D.

[95] USAC Aug. 2 Data Letter at 2

[96] *Id.*

[97] USAC Feb. 17 Letter at 1.

[98] *Id.*

provided temporary "bridge" funding to those projects with sites that will have exhausted their Pilot funding before the end of funding year 2012 (before June 30, 2013).[99]

Figure 4 - Cumulative Pilot Program Disbursements[100]

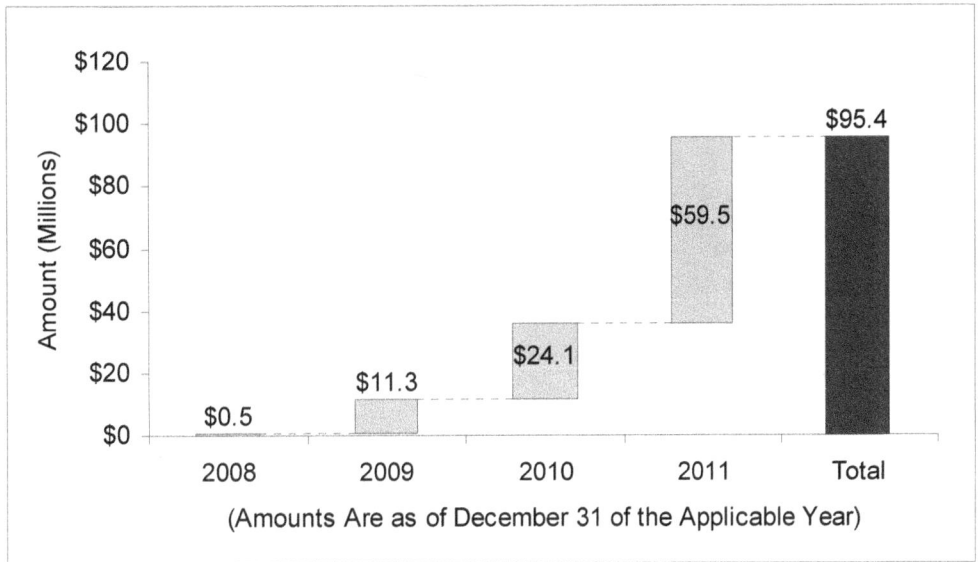

B. Geographic Coverage of Projects

34. *Interactive Map of Projects.* Currently, active Pilot projects include sites in 38 states and three territories, and many of the projects are state-wide or multi-state regional networks.[101] An interactive map showing the broadband connectivity enabled by the Pilot Program as of January 31, 2012, can be found at http://www.fcc.gov/maps/rural-health-care-pilot-program. The map shows the health care provider locations that have received commitments for Pilot Program funding, and for each location (via mouse-over), the speed of the connection, the type of health care provider, and the urban or rural status of the health care provider.

---

[99] *See supra* para. 22; *see also Bridge Funding Order.*

[100] USAC May 4 Data Letter at 3.

[101] *Id.*, App. A; *see also* Appendix A to this Staff Report.

Figure 5 – Map of Pilot Projects[102]

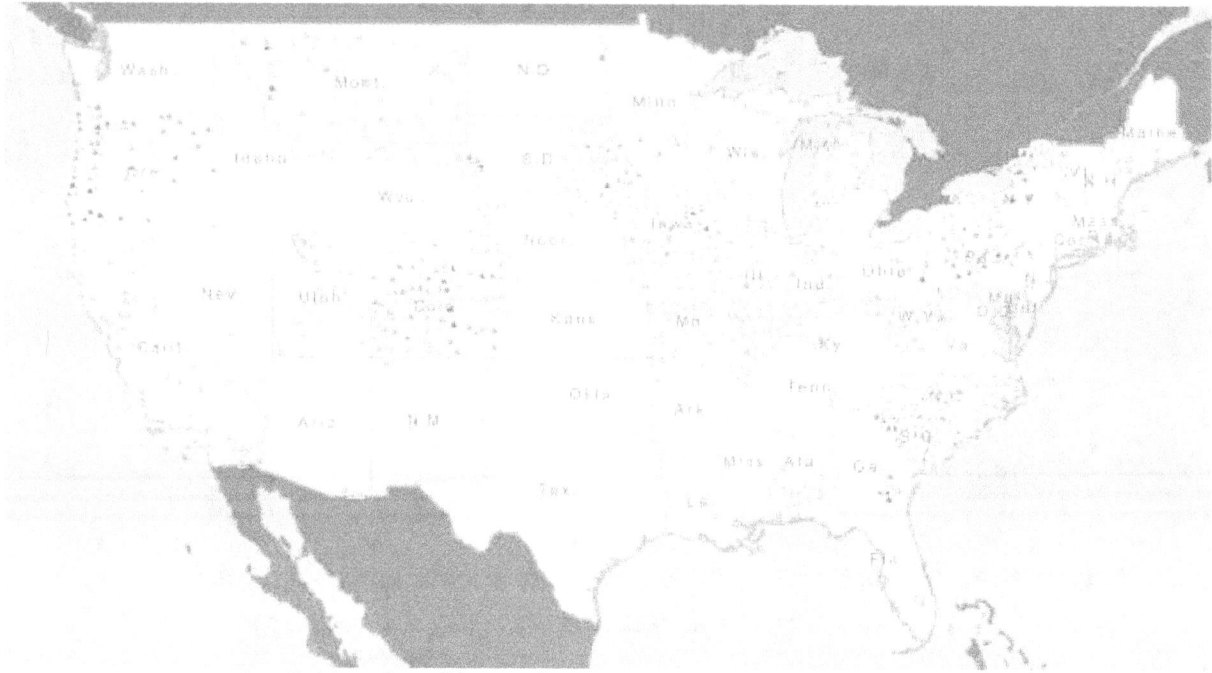

(available at http://fcc.gov/maps/rural-health-care-pilot-program)

35. Active pilot projects currently include health care providers in the 38 states listed in Appendix A and in the territories of Guam, American Samoa, and in the Northern Mariana Islands. Of the 11 states without Pilot project participants, five are almost entirely urban (Maryland, Delaware, New Jersey, Rhode Island, and Connecticut).[103] No projects applied from Oklahoma or Idaho.[104] Massachusetts was not awarded a Pilot project.[105] Projects in Kansas and Florida withdrew, one due to an inability to meet competitive bidding requirements (Kansas) and the other because it obtained

---

[102] Rural health care providers participating in Pilot Program networks are shown in green; urban health care providers are shown in red. The graphic is intended to illustrate the coverage of Pilot Program commitments as of January 31, 2012, and has two limitations that do not exist in the online map. First, the graphic does not show Alaska, Hawaii, and U.S. territories (for space reasons). Second, again due to space reasons, the graphic does not include a marker for all health care providers who had received commitments as of January 31, 2012. The interactive map allows viewers to zoom in on different areas of the country to fully see all health care providers receiving support in a particular area.

[103] These states also have no federally designated rural health clinics or critical access hospitals. *See* Critical Access Hospitals in the Rural Health Care Program. *See* Letter from Craig Davis, Vice President of Rural Health Care, USAC, to Julie Veach, Chief, Wireline Competition Bureau, WC Docket No. 02-60 (filed Jul. 19, 2012) (attachment) (USAC Critical Access Hospitals Report).

[104] *See 2007 Pilot Program Selection Order,* 21 FCC Rcd at 20426-28, App. A (listing Pilot Program applicants). We note that Oklahoma has a robust state universal service program for the communications needs of rural health care providers. *See* Oklahoma Corporation Commission, Public Utility Division, Universal Service Fund, *available at* http://www.occeweb.com/pu/OUSF/OUSF.htm (last visited April 2, 2012); *see also* Federal Communications Commission Response to United States House of Representatives Committee on Energy and Commerce, Universal Service Fund Data Request 2: States with a Statewide Universal Service Fund, at 6, 10 (dated June 22, 2011), *available at* http://republicans.energycommerce.house.gov/Media/file/PDFs/2011usf/ResponsetoQuestion2.pdf.

[105] Massachusetts had one application, which was denied in part because the application sought support "focused not for a network dedicated to telehealth, but instead for a network for use by public schools, community colleges, and commercial firms." *See 2007 Pilot Program Selection Order,* 22 FCC Rcd at 20390, para. 57.

Recovery Act funding for its project (Florida).[106] Finally, projects in Mississippi and Washington State failed to meet the June 30, 2011 deadline for submitting their first funding commitment requests.[107]

C. Rural/Urban Composition of Projects

36. *Rural versus Urban Sites.* As discussed above, in the Commission's Primary Rural Health Care Program, only "rural" health care providers within the meaning of the Commission's rules may receive funding.[108] By contrast, in the Pilot Program, the Commission has specifically allowed projects to include urban health care providers, as long as the urban HCPs are not-for-profit or public, and as long as there is a more than a *de minimis* representation of rural HCPs in the project.[109]

37. As of January 2012, approximately $139 million, or about 65 percent of committed funds, had been committed to health care providers in rural locations.[110] Approximately $78 million, or about 35 percent, of committed funds had been committed to health care providers located in urban areas. [111] This 35 percent figure attributed to urban locations, however, is likely overstated because shared equipment and services are often attributed to urban locations, even though the shared equipment and services are used by all the network sites.[112] In addition to network design studies, "shared" equipment and services (*i.e.,* equipment and services that benefit the entire network and not just one site) would include switches, routers, and firewalls that are located at data centers or other facilities of lead entities that often are located in urban areas.[113]

---

[106] USAC May 4 Data Letter at 2.

[107] *Id.*

[108] 47 U.S.C. § 254(h)(1)(A).

[109] *See generally 2006 Pilot Program Order,* 21 FCC Rcd at 1111, para. 3; *2007 Pilot Program Selection Order,* 22 FCC Rcd at 20421, para. 120.

[110] USAC May 4 Data Letter at 3. Whether a health care provider is "rural" depends on where it is located in relationship to any Core Based Statistical Area (CBSA). An area located outside of any CBSA is rural. However, areas within a CBSA can be rural, depending on the characteristics of the census tract where it is located. *See 2004 Second Report and Order and Further Notice,* 19 FCC Rcd at 24619-20, para. 12; *see also 2006 Pilot Program Order*, 21 FCC Rcd at 11116, para. 16 (stating that the Commission will not accept proposals to participate in the Rural Health Care Pilot Program that do not have more than a *de minimis* number of rural health care providers). The term "urban," used here to mean outside "rural" areas as defined by the Commission, may also include sites located in areas that are relatively sparsely populated, but do not qualify as "rural."

[111] USAC May 4 Data Letter at 3.

[112] USAC May 30 Data Letter at 2.

[113] *Id.*

Figure 6 – Urban/Rural Composition of Each Pilot Project[114]

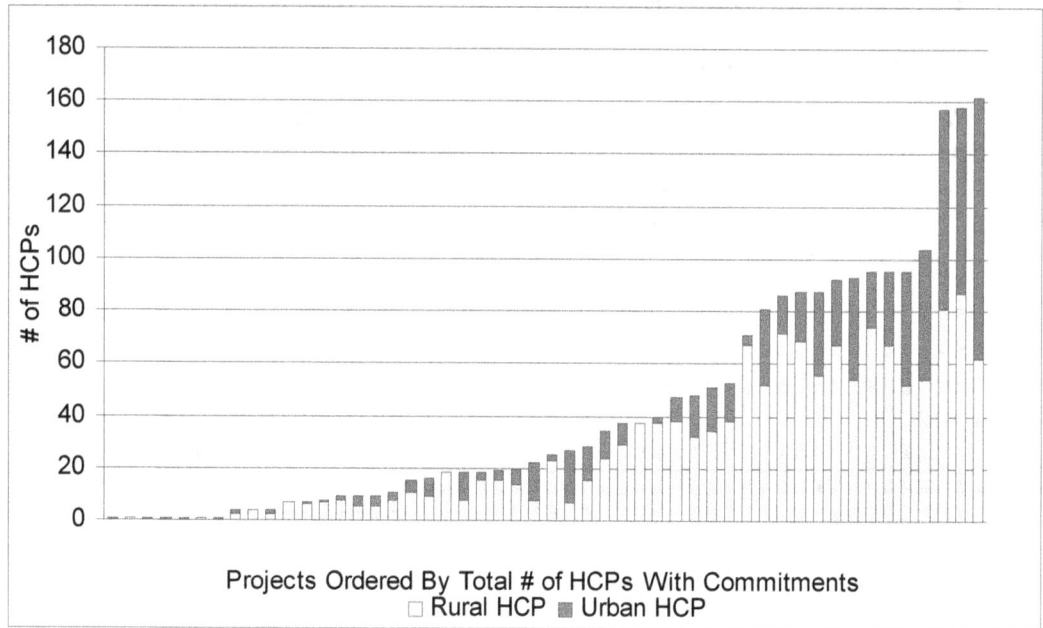

38. Figure 6 above shows the number of rural and urban health care providers participating in each Pilot project, ranging from the smallest projects to the largest projects. As shown in the figure, most projects are made up predominantly of rural health care providers and as of January 31, 2012, only six projects do not have an urban provider in their network.[115] A few projects are large-scale, statewide networks, consistent with the *2006 Pilot Program Order* (which encouraged such networks).[116] The largest five projects (at the far right) are statewide networks in West Virginia, Colorado, Oregon, South Carolina, and California, as shown in the health care provider map located at http://fcc.gov/maps/rural-health-care-pilot-program. Due to their statewide footprints, which include densely populated regions in their networks, these networks have larger percentages of health care providers located in urban areas than do smaller, regional networks that focus their coverage on specific rural areas within a state. Approximately 35 percent, or 733, of the 2,107 health care providers that had received funding commitments in the Pilot Program as of January 31, 2012, are classified as urban.[117]

D.   Types of Health Care Providers Participating in Projects

39. *Types of Health Care Providers in Projects.* Section 254(h)(7)(B) of Act identifies the types of health care providers eligible to participate in the Commission's rural health care program: not-for-profit hospitals;[118] rural health clinics; community mental health centers; community health centers of

---

[114] USAC Aug. 9 Data Letter at App. E.

[115] USAC Aug. 2 Data Letter at 2.

[116] *2006 Pilot Program Order,* 21 FCC Rcd 11111, para. 16; *2007 Pilot Program Selection Order,* 22 FCC Rcd at 20370, para. 24.

[117] USAC June 27 Data Letter at 1. The mix of rural and urban providers has remained largely consistent since January 2012. *See* USAC Aug. 2 Data Letter at 3 (noting that as of July 19, 2012, urban providers make up 33.02% of Pilot sites).

[118] In 2003, the Commission determined that dedicated emergency rooms of rural for-profit hospitals qualified as "public" health care providers under section 254(h)(1)(A) of the Act, which makes "non-profit" *or* "public" health care providers eligible for rural health care support. The Commission held that dedicated emergency departments in

(continued . . .)

health centers providing health care to migrants; local health departments or agencies; post-secondary educational institutions offering health care instructions, teaching hospitals or medical schools; and consortia of the above. As depicted in Figure 7, of these categories, 773 (37 percent) of Pilot participants who have received commitments as of January 2012 are hospitals, 547 (26 percent) are rural health clinics (or the urban equivalent), 309 are community/migrant health centers (15 percent), and 318 are community mental health centers (15 percent).[119]

Figure 7 – Number of HCPs Receiving Funding Commitments[120]

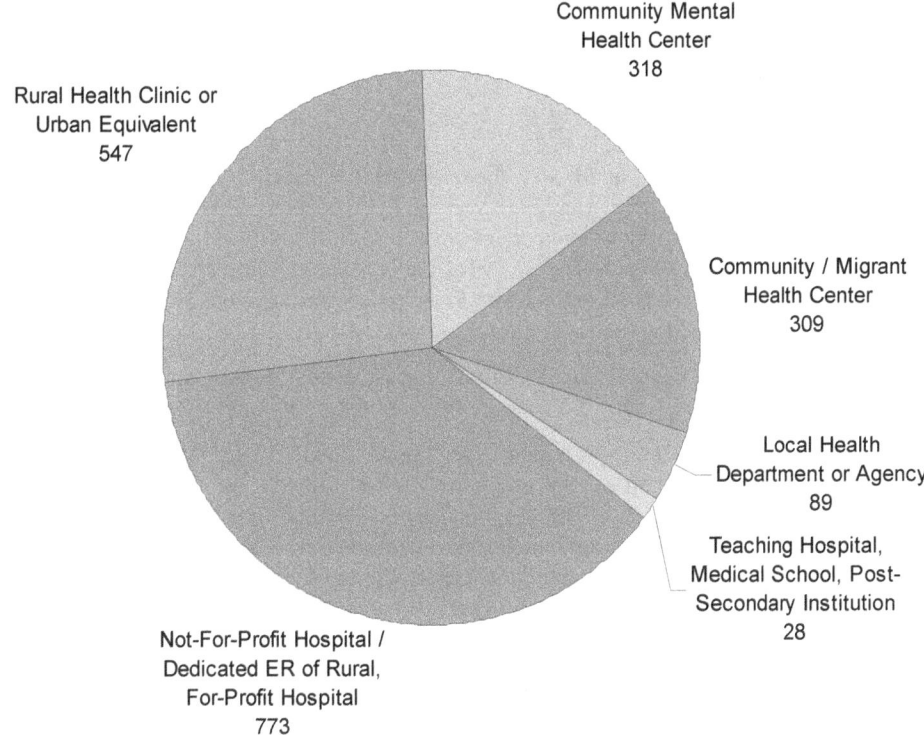

40. As noted above, as of January 2012, USAC had verified the eligibility of approximately 5,475 health care providers participating in Pilot Program networks, and issued Pilot Program funding

(. . . continued from previous page) ──────────────────────────────
for-profit hospitals are "public" health care providers because they are required, under the Emergency Medical Treatment and Labor Act to provide medical screening examinations to all patients who present themselves and to stabilize or arrange for appropriate transfer of those patients with emergency conditions. *2003 Order and Further Notice*, 18 FCC Rcd at 24553-54, para. 13. In addition, the Commission also held that dedicated emergency departments in for-profit rural hospitals constitute "rural health clinics" because they typically provide the types of medical services often provided in traditional health clinics and, in many instances, are the only health care providers in rural areas serving the medical needs of the community. *Id.* As a practical matter, however, broadband purchasing decisions for a hospital's emergency room are likely to take place in the broader context of broadband purchasing decisions for the hospital as a whole. Therefore, solely for purposes of analyzing the results of the Pilot Program in this Report, the staff has included data on the dedicated emergency rooms of for-profit hospitals within the "not-for-profit hospital" category.

[119] USAC Aug. 9 Data Letter at App. F.

[120] *Id.*

commitments to more than 2,100 health care providers.[121] Most projects included a wide range of HCP types.[122] The Pilot Program provides funding for a number of "safety net provider" health care sites, including many Critical Access Hospitals, Rural Health Clinics, and Federally Qualified Health Centers.[123] Several Pilot projects include health care provider sites that are located on Tribal lands or that serve Indian populations.[124]

41. The Commission also permits Pilot projects to include health care provider sites that are not eligible to receive funding under the rural health care program (*e.g.*, for-profit providers), so long as they pay for their own connections.[125] Nineteen projects have reported a total of approximately 138 such ineligible health care providers that participate in their networks by paying the undiscounted cost of the connection.[126]

---

[121] USAC 2011 Annual Report at 12. At the initial application stage (Form 465), Pilot projects submitted a list of all HCPs that provided a Letter of Authority, and USAC then verified the eligibility of the HCPs. *See* Section II.C above. Only those HCPs for which eligibility has been verified may receive a funding commitment (Form 466-A). *See id.* In comparison, the Primary Program funds approximately 2,000 to 3,000 eligible health care providers annually. *See* 2010 Universal Service Monitoring Report at Table 5.2, 2011 Universal Service Monitoring Report at Table 2.22 (2,695 health care providers received Primary Program commitments in FY 2007; 2,871 in FY 2008; 3,164 in FY 2009; and 1,941 in FY 2010).

[122] *See* Appendix C (detailing the number of each HCP type that received a funding commitment as of January 31, 2012).

[123] *See* John Gale Mar. 29 Ex Parte Letter (attachments) (Centers for Medicare and Medicaid Services Fact Sheets on Critical Access Hospitals, Rural Health Clinics, and Federally Qualified Health Centers). According to the Centers for Medicare and Medicaid Services (CMS), critical access hospitals are Medicare-participating hospitals that, among other characteristics, furnish 24-hour emergency care seven days a week, are located more than 35 miles from the nearest hospital, and have an average annual length to stay of 96 hours or less per patient for acute care. Federally qualified health centers are "safety net" providers such as community health centers, public housing centers, outpatient health programs funded by the Indian Health Service, and programs serving migrants. Rural health clinics provide the services of physicians, nurse practitioners, physicians' assistants, midwives, clinical psychologists, and clinical social workers, along with services incident to those furnished by these providers. *See id.; see also* USAC Critical Access Hospitals Report at 1.

[124] These include: (1) the Southwest Telehealth Access Grid, which is a multi-state regional network in the southwestern United States; (2) the California Telehealth Network, which includes several HCP sites that serve Tribal populations; (3) the Alaska eHealth Network, which to date has received funding commitments only for network design studies; and (4) the Health Information Exchange of Montana, which serves four HCP sites on Tribal lands. *See* Letter from Jeffrey Mitchell, Counsel for Health Information Exchange of Montana, to Marlene Dortch, Secretary, FCC, WC Docket No. 02-60 (filed June 21, 2012). In addition, under the Commission's Primary program, substantial funds ($35,625,539 in 2010) go to the Indian Health Service and directly to Tribal entities to fund health care facilities located on Tribal lands or serving rural Tribal populations. USAC Aug. 2 Data Letter at 1. *See also* IHS Apr. 11 *Ex Parte* Letter at 1 (summary of discussion that the rural health care program had been useful in funding broadband connections in many tribal areas and communities). In Alaska, the average effective discount under the Primary Program is 97.89 percent, so even though there are substantial Native populations in Alaska, there may be less incentive in that state to participate in the Pilot Program, which has an 85 percent discount. USAC May 30 Data Letter at 1.

[125] *2006 Pilot Program Order*, 21 FCC Rcd at 11116, para 17 (requiring applicants to "[d]escribe how for-profit network participants will pay their fair share of network cost."); *2007 Pilot Program Selection Order*, 22 FCC Rcd at 20381-20382, para. 47 (describing how for-profit network participants on Pilot networks will pay for their fair share of the network and other costs).

[126] *See* Quarterly Report of Arkansas Telehealth Network at 17 (1 site); Quarterly Report of Colorado Health Care Connections, WC Docket No. 02-60 at Addendum A (filed Jan. 27, 2012) (5 sites); Quarterly Report of Health Information Exchange of Montana at 5 (1 site); Quarterly Report of Iowa Health Systems at 3 (2 sites); Quarterly

(continued . . .)

42. Figure 8 shows the breakdown within each HCP category of the number of rural and urban health care providers with funding commitments.

Figure 8 – Rural/Urban, by HCP Type[127]

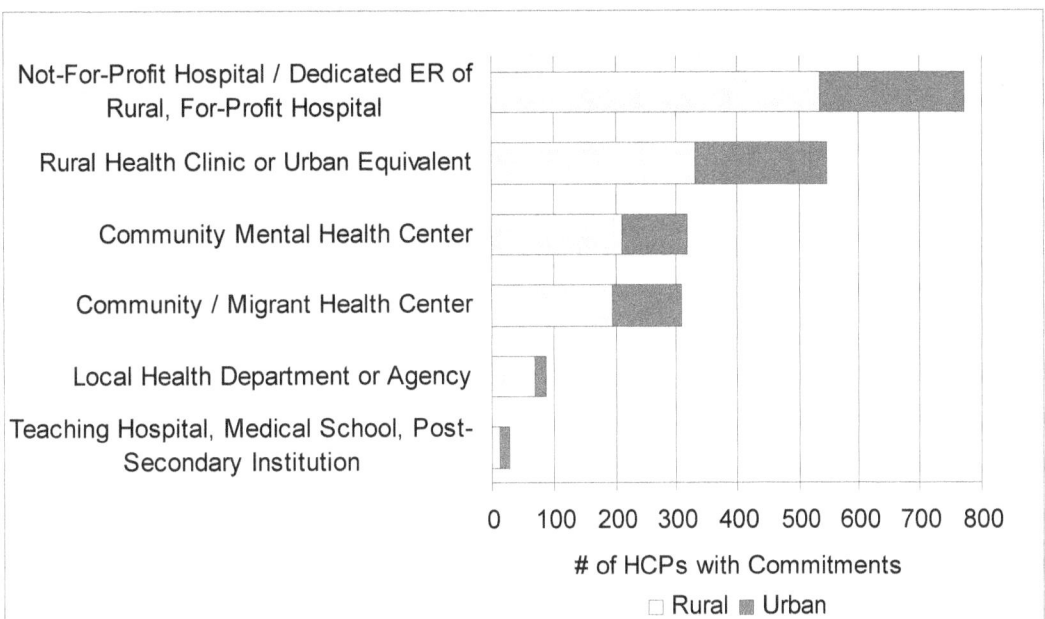

(. . . continued from previous page) ————————————————
Report of Iowa Rural Health Telecommunications Program, WC Docket No. 02-60 at 13 (filed Jan. 13, 2012) (2 sites); Quarterly Report of Michigan Public Health Institute at Appendix A (2 sites); Quarterly Report of Missouri Telehealth Network at 3, 5 (unclear how many sites); Quarterly Report of New England Telehealth Consortium, WC Docket No. 02-60 at 3-79 (filed Jan. 27, 2012) (53 sites); Quarterly Report of North Country Telemedicine Project, WC Docket No. 02-60 at 6 (filed Jan. 30, 2012) (1 site); Quarterly Report of Oregon Health Network at Attachment A (2 sites); Quarterly Report of Palmetto State Providers Network, WC Docket No. 02-60 at 3-24 (filed Jan. 30, 2012) (7 sites); Quarterly Report of Pennsylvania Mountains Healthcare Alliance, WC Docket No. 02-60 at 6 (filed Feb. 6, 2012) (1 site); Quarterly Report of Rocky Mountain HealthNet, WC Docket No. 02-60 at Addendum A (filed Jan. 27, 2012) (2 sites); Quarterly Report of Southern Ohio Healthcare Network at Addendum II (43 sites); Quarterly Report of Southwest Telehealth Access Grid (SWTAG), WC Docket No. 02-60 at Appendix A (filed Jan. 27, 2012) (5 sites); Quarterly Report of Southwest Alabama Mental Health Consortium, WC Docket No. 02-60 at 5 (filed Jan. 30, 2012) (1 site); Quarterly Report of Utah Telehealth Network, WC Docket No. 02-60 at RFP02 (filed Jan. 30, 2012) (2 sites); Quarterly Report of Western New York Rural Area Health Education Center, WC Docket No. 02-60 at 5 (filed Oct. 26, 2011) (1site); Quarterly Report of West Virginia Telehealth Alliance, WC Docket No. 02-60 at Appendix A (filed Jan. 30, 2012) (7 sites).

[127] USAC Aug. 9 Data Letter at App. H.

43. *Leadership of Projects.* USAC observes that the most successful Pilot projects have been led by universities, state entities, a hospital or medical association, or were non-profits created to advance telehealth and telemedicine initiatives in the state or region.[128] As shown below, the majority of projects designated a health care provider (or collaboration thereof) as their project coordinator.

Figure 9 – Pilot Project Coordinators[129]

Type of entity	Percentage
Health care provider	32%
Health care provider collaboration	24%
State university	18%
Multi-stakeholder collaboration	8%
Healthcare provider and university collaboration	8%
No response, likely not for profit health care consulting org.	4%
Government	4%
No response, likely health care provider collaboration	2%
Total	*100%*

E.   **Enterprise-Grade Services**

44.   The *OBI Health Care Technical Paper* found that health care providers typically need three characteristics from their broadband services – (1) bandwidth adequate to support the number and types of applications used, with two popular applications being video consultations and transfer of high-resolution medical images; (2) service quality (*i.e.*, reliability, latency, packet loss, and jitter), certain levels of which are required, for example, to support real-time, interactive video consultations; and (3) security required to allow health care providers to comply with Health Insurance Portability and Accountability Act (HIPAA) security requirements for health information.[130] The *Technical Paper* noted that in order to obtain these characteristics, most larger health care practices will require "Dedicated Internet Access" (*i.e.*, service offerings geared toward enterprise, rather than small business customers).[131] These enterprise solutions typically have several characteristics that make them suitable for many health care providers: higher guaranteed bandwidths; broader and stricter Service Level Agreements (SLAs) that can include minimum service quality guarantees; security through various means, including a dedicated connection and/or software-based solutions; and the ability to allocate bandwidth levels and prioritize certain types of traffic according to health care provider needs.[132]

45.   Not surprisingly, Pilot projects proposed dedicated, enterprise-style network architectures, designs, and topologies customized for health care purposes. Almost all projects that purchased services from third parties for their networks chose to obtain primarily Ethernet or MPLS-enabled services and to obtain customized arrangements with service providers to meet the needs of their participating health care

---

[128] USAC Observations Letter at 5.

[129] Based on staff review of Pilot participant 2011-2012 quarterly reports.

[130] *See generally* Federal Communications Commission, Health Care Broadband in America, Early Analysis and A Path Forward (August 2010) (*OBI Health Care Technical Paper*).

[131] *OBI Health Care Technical Paper* at 8.

[132] *Id.*

providers.[133] Furthermore, many of these projects obtained plant or infrastructure upgrades from their service provider as part of project implementation.[134] For example:

- Oregon Health Network (OHN) states that it was able to obtain high service level requirements which, combined with a single point of peering for all vendors and an OHN Network Operations Center that provides 24/7/365 monitoring of all connections, "proved to be a game-changer for health care providers looking to make the jump from siloed health care delivery systems of the past to the future integrated, coordinated and patient centered care models of the future."[135] OHN's network design "allows for the quick adoption and use of telehealth and health IT administrative applications to run over the network with minimum barriers."[136]

- Similarly, the North Carolina Telehealth Network (NCTN) is a private network with a connection to the public Internet and Internet2, which provides connectivity beginning at 10 Mbps. NCTN provides more reliability and better latency control for video-based and other applications that need high reliability (*e.g.,* remote ICU monitoring). Thus, NCTN's network is able to serve public health agencies, which are core responders in emergency response situations and need access to a network that will be available in emergency response situations. The NCTN network also provides dual redundancy and allows members to communicate with each other without crossing the public Internet.[137]

- The Sanford Health Collaboration and Communication Channel (with sites in South Dakota, Iowa, and Minnesota) also used Pilot funding to upgrade from T-1 lines to Ethernet services. Sanford stated that upgrading to Ethernet helped it to roll out electronic health records, because T-1s were not adequate for this purpose.[138]

---

[133] USAC June 27 Data Letter at 1. The Telecommunications Industry Association notes that Ethernet "provides much faster speeds than other technologies at substantially lower costs" and "is a cost-effective technology for companies with high bandwidth needs" who need to connect to data centers, make other point-to-point connections, or with multiple locations. Over fiber networks, carrier Ethernet can provide speeds of up to 10 Gbps at a much lower cost than legacy technologies, although Ethernet services are also available over copper facilities. *See* Telecommunications Industry Association, *2012 ICT Market Review and Forecast*, at 3-8, 3-38, 3-42 (*TIA 2012 Market Review and Forecast*). MPLS is a network protocol that allows providers to create a single integrated network infrastructure that can be used to provide multiple services to the enterprise customer. *See Universal Service Contribution Methodology; A National Broadband Plan For Our Future,* WC Docket No. 06-122, GN Docket No. 09-51, Further Notice of Proposed Rulemaking, 27 FCC Rcd 5357, 5380, para. 41 (2012). TIA notes that carriers are converting to MPLS in their core networks to facilitate IP transport, and that MPLS-enabled networks can establish different classes of services and offer guarantees of service without dedicated circuits. MPLS-enabled networks can also provide the security of virtual private circuits with the any-to-any connectivity of router-based networks. Furthermore, carriers charge less for MPLS than for other technologies because the costs for provisioning and supporting it are lower. *TIA 2012 Market Review and Forecast* at 3-8, 3-40.

Of course, projects that chose to construct their own networks also had the ability to control service quality and reliability over the network. *See, e.g.,* Pilot Conference Call Mar. 26 *Ex Parte* Letter (WNYRAHEC *et al.*) at 1.

[134] *See* USAC Aug. 2 Data Letter at 3.

[135] OHN Feb. 28 *Ex Parte* Letter at 2.

[136] *Id.*

[137] Pilot Conference Call Mar. 13 Ex Parte Letter (PMHA et al.) at 2; Quarterly Report of the North Carolina Telehealth Network, WC Docket No. 02-60, at 28-9 (filed Jan. 31, 2012).

[138] Pilot Conference Call Mar. 26 *Ex Parte* Letter (WNYRAHEC *et al.*) at 1-2.

46. In addition, over 20 Pilot projects have high-bandwidth connections to other health care provider networks through either Internet2 or National LambdaRail, though many do not rely on Pilot funding for those connections.[139]

F.   Self-Construction versus Services Purchased from Third Parties

47. As noted above, the Pilot Program allows participants to build or lease their networks.[140] Initially, in the 2006 *Pilot Program Order*, the Commission provided support through the Rural Health Care Pilot Program for public and non-profit health care providers to construct and own their networks.[141] This was later clarified to allow projects also to subscribe to leased transmission services as a means of creating their broadband networks.[142] A majority of Pilot projects have chosen to purchase broadband services rather than construct and operate a broadband network themselves. Only eight projects used Pilot Program support for construction, and only two constructed their entire networks.[143] Instead, most have purchased services, with a significant number using the funding to purchase long term prepaid leases or indefeasible rights of use (IRUs).[144] As of January 2012, nearly 80 percent of funding commitments were attributable to purchased services, as shown in Figures 10(a) and 10(b).

---

[139] *See* USAC May 4 Data Letter at 4. Pilot Program rules allowed projects to connect to Internet2 and National LambdaRail without requiring projects to go through the competitive bidding process. *See Rural Health Care Support Mechanism*, WC Docket No. 02-60, Order on Reconsideration, 22 FCC Rcd 2555 (2007) (*Pilot Program Order on Reconsideration*). Based on available data, several projects have availed themselves of this opportunity. The following Pilot projects have requested and received funding commitments from USAC for their Internet2 connections (no projects have sought funding for membership to the National LambdaRail network): California Telehealth Network, Iowa Health Systems, North Carolina Telehealth Network, St. Joseph's Hospital and Texas Health Information Network Collaborative. USAC May 4 Data Letter at 4.

[140] *See supra* n.30 and accompanying text.

[141] *2006 Pilot Program Order*, 21 FCC Rcd at 11115, paras. 3, 14.

[142] *See 2007 Pilot Program Selection Order*, 22 FCC Rcd at 20397-98, para. 74 ("In the *2006 Pilot Program Order*, the Commission stated that funding provided under the Pilot Program would be used to support the costs of constructing dedicated broadband networks that connect health care providers in a state or region. . . Further, to the extent that a selected participant subscribes to carrier-provided transmission services. . . in lieu of deploying its own broadband network and access to advanced telecommunications and information services, the costs for subscribing to such facilities and services are eligible") (citing *2006 Pilot Program Order*, 21 FCC Rcd at 11114, para. 10).

[143] Projects that used Pilot Program funds to construct and own their networks entirely include Northeast Ohio Regional Health Information Organization and Rural Nebraska Healthcare Network. The Iowa Rural Health Telecommunications Program, Illinois Rural HealthNet Consortium, Health Information Exchange of Montana, Michigan Public Health Institute, St. Joseph's Hospital and West Virginia Telehealth Alliance used Pilot Program funds to construct and own parts of their networks. USAC May 4 Data Letter at 3, App. D.

[144] USAC Observations Letter at 7-8. *See* Section V.C. *infra,* which discusses the reasons cited by some Pilot projects for relying on purchased services rather than constructing and owning their networks. For example, the Colorado Telehealth Network stated that it was able to include more providers on its network through purchasing services than if it chose to construct and own its network. Colorado Feb. 28 *Ex Parte* Letter at 2. Oregon Health Network also explained that it successfully created its network by implementing a multi-vendor leased line network. OHN Feb. 28 *Ex Parte* Letter at 1.

Figure 10(a) – Pilot Funding Commitments for Self-Construction versus Third Party Services (Millions)[145]

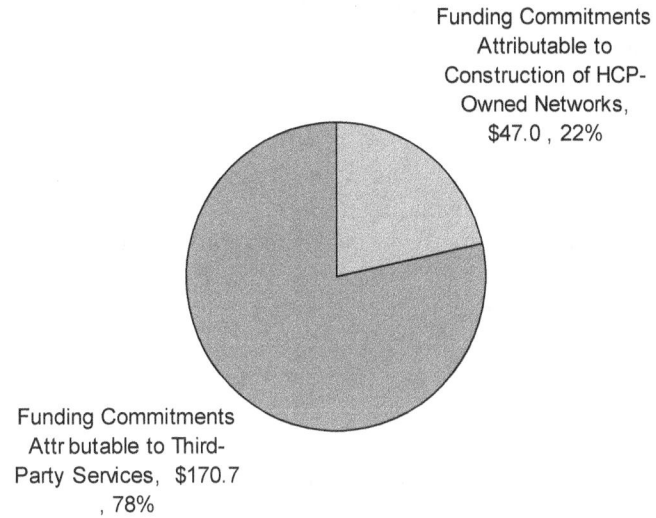

Funding Commitments Attributable to Construction of HCP-Owned Networks, $47.0 , 22%

Funding Commitments Attributable to Third-Party Services, $170.7 , 78%

Figure 10(b) – Breakdown of Pilot Funding Commitments for Construction Versus Services[146]

Funding Commitments Attributable to Construction of HCP-Owned Networks	Amount (Millions)
Infrastructure/Outside Plant (Engineering & Construction)	$35.2
Network Equipment (including Engineering & Installation)	$10.3
Network Mgmt/Maint/Operations (not captured elsewhere)	$1.5
Subtotal	**$47.0**
Funding Commitments Attributable to Third-Party Services	
Leased/Tariffed Facilities or Services	$156.6
Network Design	$1.9
Network Equipment (including Engineering & Installation)	$9.0
Network Mgmt/Maint/Operations (not captured elsewhere)	$2.6
Internet 2/NLR/Internet	$0.6
Subtotal	**$170.7**
Total	**$217.7**

48. Although the majority of funding commitments have been for third-party services, Pilot Projects, where necessary, have used construction funding to extend connectivity to over 400 health care provider locations.[147] For example, several projects have used Pilot Program funds to construct and own last-mile connections to HCPs or to create parts of their network where there was no other competitive option. St. Joseph's Hospital states that it found constructing and owning part of its private fiber

---

[145] USAC Aug. 2 Data Letter at 3-4 (providing funding commitments for construction and leased services as of Jan. 31, 2012).

[146] *Id.*

[147] USAC May 4 Data Letter at 3.

network helped it control costs and ensure its long-term success.[148] It states that purchasing the 10 Gbps connection it needed to move medical images would have been cost-prohibitive. Owning its own facilities is less expensive, gives it more control of its network, and provides better quality and reliability of service.[149] At least one project indicates that the ability to construct facilities in the absence of a suitable competitive bid may have had some constraining effect on prices bid for projects.[150]

49. The two projects that relied entirely on construction each received $9 million in funding commitments for construction to connect, in total, approximately 94 health care providers.[151] For projects that are "partially constructed," funding commitments for construction, on a per-project basis as of January 30, 2012, ranged from $350,000 to $7 million.[152] Very roughly, $35 million in construction commitments to over 230 health care providers equates to approximately $150,000 per health care provider.[153] Assuming a life of 15 years for constructed facilities, this equates to an annualized cost of about $2.3 million a year to the Fund to serve over 230 health care providers, or a cost of approximately $830 per month per health care provider.[154] By comparison, in funding year 2010, it cost on average approximately $560 per month for the Primary Program to fund circuits in the 1.5 to 3 Mbps range.[155] Thus, based on Pilot commitments as of January 31, 2012, it appears that the self-construction option, if chosen and requested by Pilot Projects after competitive bidding, provides Pilot project health care providers with higher-bandwidth services at only an incrementally higher cost to the fund (less than $1 million per year[156]) than the current Primary Program. Moreover, health care providers' prices for the higher bandwidth are generally comparable to, or less than, the prices for lower speed services currently being ordered through the Primary Program, as further discussed below in Section III.G.

50. *Equipment Purchase.* Unlike the Primary Program, the Pilot Program provides support to purchase equipment such as servers, routers, firewalls, switches, and other devices or equipment

---

[148] Pilot Conference Call Mar. 26 *Ex Parte* Letter (WNYRAHEC *et al*) at 1.

[149] *Id.*

[150] HIEM Sept. 22 *Ex* Parte Letter at 2. *See also* Comments of Health Information Exchange of Montana, WC Docket No. 02-60, at 10-11 (filed May 25, 2012) (HIEM May 25 Comments).

[151] The two projects that have relied entirely on construction are Rural Nebraska Healthcare Network ($9.4 million) and Northeast Ohio Regional Health Information Organization ($9.3 million). *See* USAC May 4 Data Letter at 3-4 and Appendix D; USAC June 27 Data Letter at 3 and Appendix A.

[152] These projects include Health Information Exchange of Montana ($7.4 million), Illinois Rural HealthNet Consortium ($2.8 million), Iowa Rural Health Telecommunications Program ($5.1 million), Michigan Public Health Institute ($410,000), St. Joseph's Hospital ($350,000), and West Virginia Telehealth Alliance ($465,000). *See* USAC May 4 Data Letter at 3-4 and App. D; USAC June 27 Data Letter at 3 and App. A.

[153] USAC estimates that of the eight Pilot projects that have used funds to construct and own parts of their networks, 230 health care providers have received funding commitments to fund construction. *See* USAC May 4 Data Letter at 3.

[154] Note that these figures are estimates and do not account for inflation or other factors.

[155] *See infra* Fig. 13(b).

[156] Assuming that it costs $560 per month on average under the Primary Program to support a single health care provider at the 1.5 to 3 Mbps level, the cost to serve 230 health care providers for 12 months would be $1.5456 million. When compared with the estimated annualized cost of $2.3 million a year to serve over 230 health care providers in the Pilot Program using self-constructed facilities, the difference is approximately $0.76 million.

necessary for the broadband connection.[157] Commitments for network equipment in the Pilot Program (including engineering and installation) were approximately $19.3 million for 698 health care providers in 25 projects as of January 2012.[158] In the Pilot Program, unlike in Primary Program, RHC support also can be used to upgrade equipment and increase bandwidth. For example, if it is necessary for a Pilot project to upgrade an existing HCP circuit, Pilot Program rules allow the project to receive funding for both the higher bandwidth circuit and the equipment necessary to make it operational, whereas the Primary Program would only provide funding for the higher bandwidth circuit.[159] USAC notes that because health care specialists are primarily located in urban areas, networks are typically designed in a way that results in the urban center being the "hub" of the network.[160] In order for the urban entity to act as a "hub" for the network, equipment such as routers, firewalls, servers, and switches are necessary. Because urban HCPs are natural hubs for telemedicine networks and were allowed to receive funding for equipment, the Pilot Program effectively lowered the cost of creating health care broadband networks with an urban center as the hub.[161]

51. *IRUs and Prepaid Leases.* The Pilot Program did not restrict the form of agreement that health care providers could enter into with vendors for projects funded by the program.[162] Some projects have chosen to build their networks by purchasing indefeasible rights of use (IRUs) or long-term prepaid leases, as shown below.[163] A key benefit of such long-term arrangements is that they allow health care providers to "scale up" bandwidth as their needs increase, as shown below. They also can yield lower prices and can provide longer-term price stability for health care providers.[164] These arrangements also may provide vendors the incentive to deploy broadband connections where they do not exist, or to upgrade current facilities to higher bandwidths.

---

[157] *2007 Pilot Program Selection Order*, 22 FCC Rcd at 20397-98, para. 74. *See also* USAC Observations Letter at 6-7 (explaining that unlike Primary Program participants, Pilot Program participants could use RHC support to purchase and upgrade their equipment if necessary).

[158] USAC May 4 Data Letter at 3; USAC Aug. 2 Data Letter at 3-4.

[159] *See* USAC Observations Letter at 6-7.

[160] USAC Observations Letter at 5.

[161] *Id.*; *see also* Section V.B. (discussing shortage of specialists in rural areas, and the importance of urban centers for providing specialist care in the context of telemedicine).

[162] *See 2010 NPRM*, 25 FCC Rcd at 9395, para. 55.

[163] An IRU is an indefeasible right to use facilities for a certain period of time that is commensurate with the remaining useful life of the asset, usually 20 years. The IRU confers on the grantee the vestiges of ownership, and is customarily used in the communications industry. It usually requires a large upfront payment, generally priced as a certain amount (depending on market rates) per mile or per fiber mile. *2010 NPRM*, 25 FCC Rcd at 9395-96, para. 56. In comparison, a "prepaid lease" is simply a lease with a single large upfront payment, rather than regular recurring payments.

[164] *See* Pilot Conference Call Mar. 24 *Ex Parte* Letter (AEN et al.) at 1 (explaining that the Pilot project provided economic incentive to bring broadband to the eastern shore of Virginia); USAC Observations Letter at 4.

Figure 11 – Projects Using IRU/ Prepaid Leases[165]

Project	Commitment Amount	Type of IRU/ Lease	Term	Maximum Bandwidths Available
Health Information Exchange of Montana	$108,522.97	Prepaid Lease	2 years	100 Mbps to 1 Gbps
Rural Western and Central Maine Broadband Initiative	$615,468.01	IRU	10 years	45 Mbps, 100 Mbps, 1 Gbps
Iowa Rural Health Telecommunications Program	$1,240,789.10	IRU	20 years	1 Gbps
Rural Nebraska Healthcare Network	$3,870,494.55	Prepaid Lease	15 years	100 Mbps, 1 Gbps
Michigan Public Health Institute	$5,517,313.92	IRU	20 years	1 Gbps
Iowa Health System	$6,833,296.95	IRU	15 years	10 Mbps, 30 Mbps, 100 Mbps
Illinois Rural HealthNet Consortium	$9,313,979.85	IRU	10 to 20 years	100 Mbps, 1 Gbps, 10 Gbps
Southern Ohio Healthcare Network	$15,746,105.60	Prepaid Lease	20 years	5 Mbps to 1 Gbps
Total	$43,245,970.95			

G.   Bandwidth of Services Purchased

52. The National Broadband Plan estimated that the minimum bandwidth required to support deployment of Health IT applications is 4 Mbps for single physician practices,[166] 10 Mbps for small providers (2-5 physicians),[167] 25 Mbps for clinics and large physician practices (5-25 physicians), and 100 Mbps for hospitals.[168] In addition, an August 2010 Commission staff analysis suggested that health care providers need at least 10 Mbps to achieve full functionality of high-definition video conferencing for health care purposes.[169]

53. The focus of the Pilot Program was to encourage health care providers to obtain access to *broadband* connections. The data shows that HCPs do in fact use the Pilot funding to obtain high bandwidth connections, with 80 percent purchasing connections above 3 Mbps and 69 percent purchasing 10 Mbps or greater connections.[170] In the Primary Program, by contrast, all telecommunications services are supported, whether or not considered "broadband."[171] The vast majority of connections in the Primary Program are relatively low bandwidth connections (approximately 80 percent are 3 Mbps or less).[172] Figure 12 below shows the bandwidth levels that

---

[165] USAC Aug. 9 Data Letter at App. I.

[166] We note that in certain rural areas, it is possible that rural health clinics and other small health care providers may only have a single medical professional.

[167] This category includes small primary care practices (2-4 physicians), nursing homes, and rural health centers (~5 physicians). *See* National Broadband Plan at 210-211.

[168] *See id.* The *National Broadband Plan* also recommended that academic/large medical centers receive at least 1 Gbps to support the deployment of Health IT. *See also OBI Health Care Technical Paper* at 6.

[169] *OBI Health Care Technical Paper* at 5; *see also* USAC Needs Assessment at 3.

[170] *See* Fig. 12.

[171] *See* 47 C.F.R. § 54.601(c).

[172] *See* Fig. 13(a).

health care providers in the Pilot Program were able to obtain for services purchased from third parties (services with recurring charges).[173] For purpose of comparison, Figure 12 shows the bandwidth levels obtained by health care providers in the Primary Program in Funding Year 2010, the last year for which full funding year information is available.[174]

Figure 12 – Pilot HCPs, By Bandwidth Tier[175]

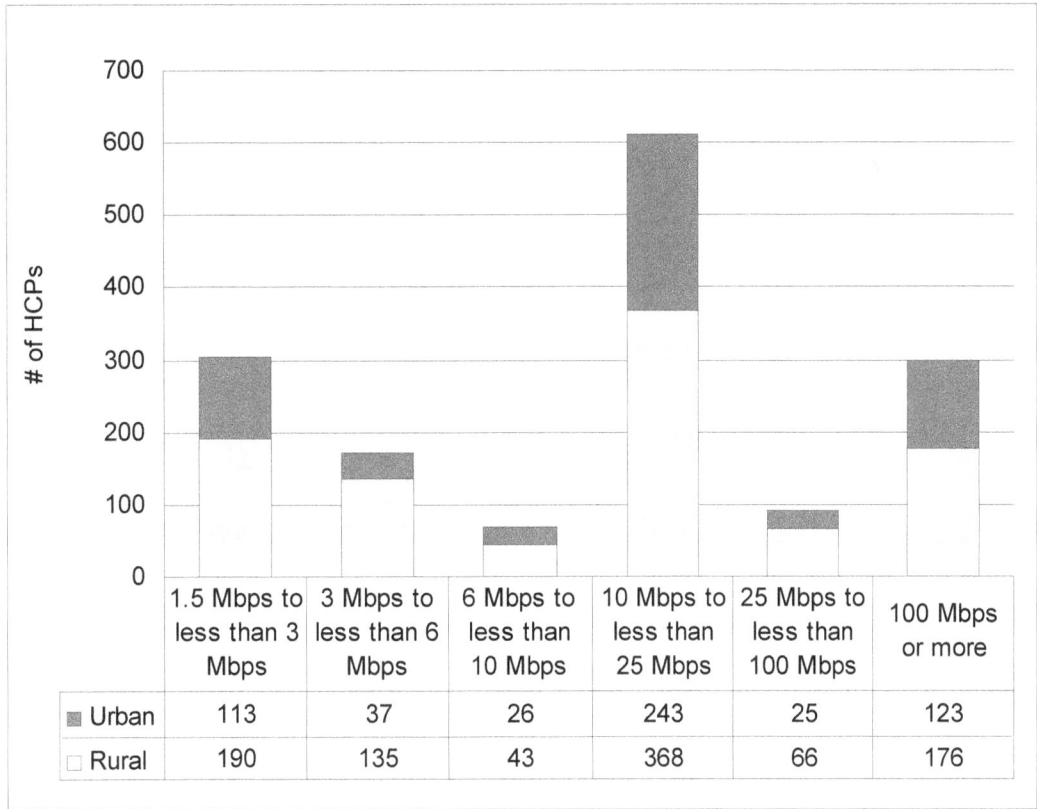

	1.5 Mbps to less than 3 Mbps	3 Mbps to less than 6 Mbps	6 Mbps to less than 10 Mbps	10 Mbps to less than 25 Mbps	25 Mbps to less than 100 Mbps	100 Mbps or more
Urban	113	37	26	243	25	123
Rural	190	135	43	368	66	176

---

[173] This figure does not include arrangements requiring large, up-front payments and a long-term commitment – *i.e.,* prepaid leases and IRUs.

[174] Funding Year 2010 covers the period from July 1, 2010 to June 30, 2011.

[175] USAC Aug. 9 Data Letter at App. J.

Figure 13(a) – Primary Program Circuits (minus Alaska) by Bandwidth Tier[176]

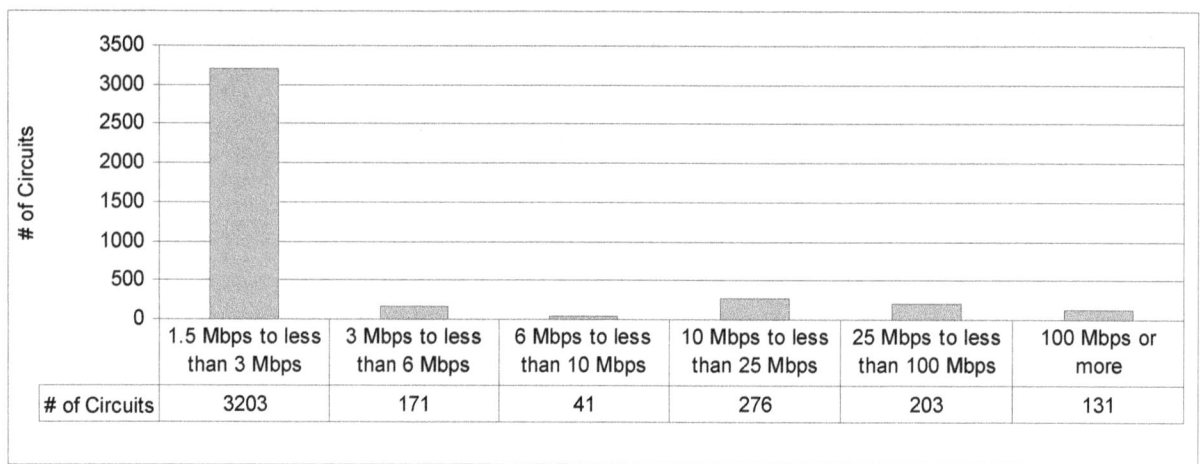

# of Circuits	1.5 Mbps to less than 3 Mbps	3 Mbps to less than 6 Mbps	6 Mbps to less than 10 Mbps	10 Mbps to less than 25 Mbps	25 Mbps to less than 100 Mbps	100 Mbps or more
# of Circuits	3203	171	41	276	203	131

Figure 13(b) – Primary Program (minus Alaska) Average Monthly Recurring Cost by Bandwidth[177]

		Average Recurring Cost per Month		
	# Of Circuits	Primary Program Support	HCP Contribution	Total Cost
1.5 Mbps to less than 3 Mbps	3203	$564	$249	$813
3 Mbps to less than 6 Mbps	171	$678	$504	$1,181
6 Mbps to less than 10 Mbps	41	$1,686	$761	$2,447
10 Mbps to less than 25 Mbps	276	$1,548	$629	$2,177
25 Mbps to less than 100 Mbps	203	$3,414	$2,039	$5,453
100 Mbps or more	131	$4,566	$1,505	$6,070

54. As shown in Figures 13(a) and 13(b), the vast majority of Primary Program participants (all of which are rural by definition) obtain bandwidths in the T-1 (1.5 to less than 3 Mbps) range.[178] As

---

[176] USAC Aug. 9 Data Letter at App. K (explaining that the analysis includes only recurring services where the applicant requested funding based on the urban/rural differential and that the analysis excludes voice services, multi-billed circuits, and those circuits where funding was based on mileage).

[177] *Id.*

[178] Some participants may obtain multiple T-1 lines, depending on their bandwidth needs. This approach, however, has several disadvantages. For example, there are no cost savings when "scaling up" because two T-1 lines generally cost twice as much as one T-1 line. *See* NRHRC Dec. 27 *Ex Parte* Letter at 2. Furthermore, health care providers who rely on multiple T-1 lines to use higher-bandwidth applications need *each* line to provide the requisite level of service quality – if one line fails, the health care provider may not be able to use the application in a way that provides high quality medical service. For example, if a remote diagnosis requires videoconferencing *and* image transmission, and a health care provider uses a separate T-1 line for each application, then the diagnosis cannot take place unless both T-1 lines function properly.

shown in Figure 12, in contrast, only about a quarter of Pilot Program health care providers opted for such lower-bandwidth lines; the remainder has received commitments for 3 Mbps or more, with nearly 60 percent of providers obtaining commitments for at least 10 Mbps. As these charts show, the average bandwidth of rural HCPs participating in the Pilot Program is significantly higher than the bandwidth of rural HCPs in the Primary Program.

Figure 14 – Bandwidths by HCP Type[179]

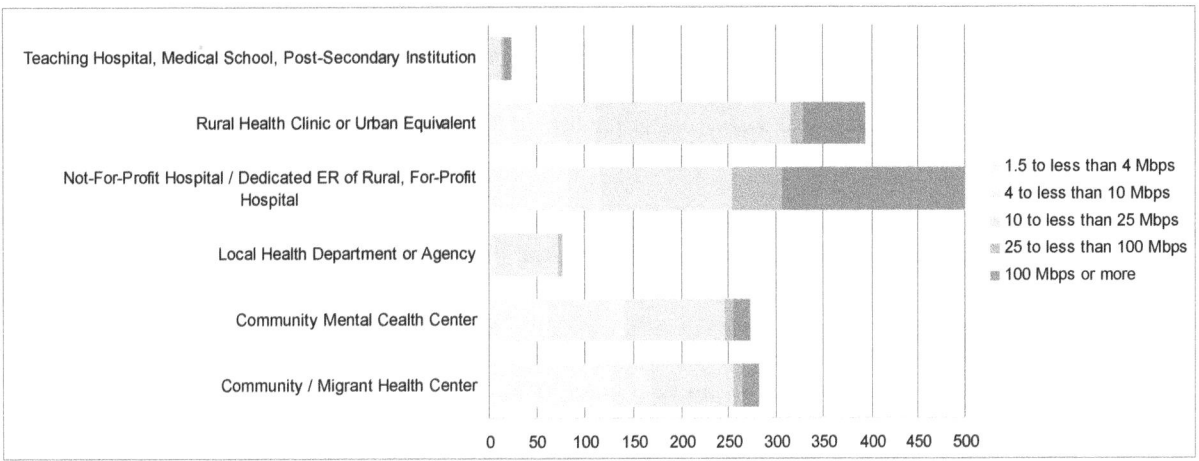

55. Figure 14 shows the bandwidths obtained by HCPs in the Pilot Program, according to the bandwidth tiers suggested in the *National Broadband Plan* (4 Mbps for single physician practices, 10 Mbps for small providers, 25 Mbps for clinics and large physician practices, and 100 Mbps for hospitals).[180] As would be expected, hospitals tend to obtain more of the higher bandwidth connections, though many clinics and health centers purchased 10 Mbps or more connections. Most health care providers, with the exception of community/migrant health centers, receive more than 10 Mbps under the Pilot Program and more than 70 percent of rural health care clinics receive bandwidth of at least 10 Mbps. Many not-for profit hospitals receive even faster speeds, with approximately 40 percent receiving 100 Mbps or more. The bandwidth recommended in the National Broadband Plan and in the OBI Report for various types of health care practices matches up well with the bandwidth purchased by most health care provider types in the Pilot Program.[181]

56. Finally, a key characteristic of many Pilot projects is the ability to offer their participating health care providers a variety of speeds and the ability to easily reallocate or increase bandwidth, as needed. For example, the North Carolina Telehealth Network (NCTN) provides a network throughout 55 North Carolina counties with a standard service of 10 Mbps for smaller subscribers (*e.g.,* clinics) and 100 Mbps to 1 Gbps for larger subscribers (*e.g.,* hospitals).[182] Similarly, the Palmetto State Providers Network provides a network throughout all 46 South Carolina countries with a standard service of 10 Mbps and a 1 Gbps shared backbone.[183] The Iowa Rural Health Telecommunications Program provides HCP-owned last mile connections to a local Internet access point for over 80 HCPs through Iowa, with

---

[179] USAC Aug. 9 Data Letter at App. L.

[180] *See supra* para. 52.

[181] *OBI Health Care Technical Paper* at 6.

[182] USAC Apr. 27 Site Visit Reports at 2.

[183] USAC Mar. 16 Site Visit Reports at 9.

bandwidth speeds varying from 30 Mbps to 60 Mbps depending on the needs of the local HCP.[184] Pennsylvania Mountains Healthcare Resource Development provides speeds varying from 10 Mbps to 100 Mbps depending on the needs of the HCP.[185]

H.   Reduced Cost of High Bandwidth Connections

57. Not only has the Pilot Program increased the bandwidth obtained by participating health care providers, it also has increased their broadband purchasing power. According to a 2010 survey conducted by the Government Accountability Office, nearly all Pilot participants indicated that their project would "definitely" or "probably" have entities that obtain telecommunications or Internet services that would be unaffordable without the project.[186] Projects have also reported to the Commission that "many of their healthcare participants will be able to obtain higher bandwidth for costs similar to what they were paying before the RHCPP."[187]

58. Two key differences between the Pilot Program and the Primary Program are worth noting with respect to this increase in purchasing power. First, the Pilot Program requires (and facilitates) consortium applications. Many Pilot projects report significant cost savings simply on the basis of achieving economies of scale within their consortia.[188] For example, Frontier Access to Rural Healthcare in Montana stated that its monthly recurring cost per site is "projected to be renegotiated at twenty five percent less cost than the current negotiated contract."[189] The Michigan Public Health Institute also reported achieving economies of scale, stating that its 72-site consortium has succeed in driving down costs to the extent that the cost is now "less than what the [health care providers] are currently paying for internet service."[190]

59. Second, the discount rate structure under the Pilot Program may facilitate health care providers' selection of higher-bandwidth connections (in comparison to the Primary Program). To receive a discount under the Primary Program, a rural HCP must ascertain a tariffed or publicly-available rate for the desired service in an urban area within the state, and then receives a discount equal to the difference between the urban rate and the rural rate.[191] It can be difficult to find an equivalent urban rate when the connection is greater than a T-1 (as higher bandwidth services are more likely to be subject to individually negotiated rates), which may discourage some HCPs from applying for discounts for higher bandwidth services altogether. Furthermore, the urban-rural differential (and thus the effective discount rate) can be greater for a T-1 connection than for higher bandwidth connections, which could create discentives to increase the broadband capacity of their connections under the Primary Program (*e.g.*,

---

[184] *Id.* at 13.

[185] *Id.* at 15.

[186] *GAO Report* at 43 (55 of 57 respondents indicated that if they are able to accomplish their Pilot project goals, their project "definitely" or "probably" will have entities that obtain telecommunications or Internet services that would otherwise be unaffordable).

[187] Quarterly Report of Indiana Telehealth Network, WC Docket No. 02-60, at 41 (filed Jan. 27, 2012).

[188] *See* USAC May 30 Data Letter at 3 (projects that pursue a "one vendor" solution report to USAC that their ability to negotiate price reductions improved because of the economies of scale introduced through bidding the entire project at once).

[189] Quarterly Report of Frontier Access to Rural Healthcare in Montana, WC Docket No. 02-60, at 12 (filed Jan. 12, 2012).

[190] Quarterly Report of Michigan Public Health Institute, WC Docket No. 02-60, at 31 (filed Jan. 30, 2012).

[191] *See* 47 C.F.R. § 54.605.

from a T-1 to a 10 Mbps Ethernet connection), even if the jump in bandwidth could greatly increase their ability to provide high quality health care.[192] Neither of these factors is present in the Pilot Program, which provides a uniform flat rate discount regardless of the bandwidth or service chosen.

60. Below, we provide more granular data on monthly recurring costs being paid for broadband connections in the Pilot Program, broken out by bandwidth and type of health care provider. First, Figure 15 below shows the average monthly cost for obtaining service in various bandwidth tiers (divided further to show the monthly cost to the USF and to the HCP), as well as the number of HCPs receiving services in each bandwidth tier.

Figure 15 – Pilot Project Average Monthly Recurring Cost By Connection Bandwidth[193]

Bandwidth	# of HCPs	Average Recurring Cost Per Month		
		Pilot Program Support	HCP Contribution	Total Cost
1.5 Mbps to less than 3 Mbps	303	$661	$117	$778
3 Mbps to less than 6 Mbps	172	$993	$174	$1,167
6 Mbps to less than 10 Mbps	69	$1,565	$303	$1,868
10 Mbps to less than 25 Mbps	611	$1,498	$292	$1,789
25 Mbps to less than 100 Mbps	91	$1,828	$329	$2,157
100 Mbps or more	299	$1,669	$317	$1,986

61. A few trends shown in Figure 15 are worth noting:

- *1.5 to less than 3 Mbps.* While this level of service is less than ideal from a health care provider perspective,[194] the data above suggests that the Pilot Program has made a minimum level of connectivity available to even the smallest rural HCPs at an out of pocket cost of about $120/month. The total recurring average monthly cost per connection is less in the Pilot Program ($778) than in the Primary Program ($813).[195]

- *3 to less than 25 Mbps.* Most HCPs are receiving services in this middle tier, which includes the range of speeds recommended in the *National Broadband Plan* for all providers other than hospitals.[196] The cost to the Fund of supporting these services through the Pilot Program, on average, is approximately $1,000 to $1,500 per provider per month, with the cost

---

[192] *See also* NRHRC Dec. 27 *Ex Parte* Letter at 2 (observing that the incremental price steps of broadband, *i.e.*, two bonded T-1s cost twice as much as a single T-1 line, encourage rural health care providers to purchase the minimum connectivity for their networks).

[193] USAC Aug. 9 Data Letter at App. M.

[194] The FCC Omnibus Broadband Initiative Technical Paper on health care recommended that health care providers receive at least 4 Mbps. *See OBI Technical Paper* at 6.

[195] *See supra* Fig. 13(b) and 15.

[196] *National Broadband Plan* at 210-211.

to the health care provider increasing to the $175 to $300 per month range.[197] For example, the Palmetto State Providers Network states that the 85 percent discount rate enables it to provide HCPs on its network a package of 10 Mbps (5 Mbps broadband and 5 Mbps symmetrical commodity Internet) and a shared 1 Gbps Internet2 circuit with VPN and video bridge for approximately $210 per month, compared to the undiscounted rate of $400-600 that HCPs previously paid for just a T-1 (1.5 Mbps) line.[198] Another project, according to USAC, upgraded its 9.24 Mbps copper bonded T-1 service ($4,552.50 per month) with a 20 Mbps Ethernet service for a lesser cost ($3,920 per month).[199]

- *25 Mbps or greater service.* On average, it appears that the cost to the Pilot Program for higher-speed circuits is topping out at approximately $1,828 per month, and the cost to the health care provider at about $329 per month.[200] Pricing for higher-bandwidth circuits may be influenced by two factors: (1) what health care providers can afford to, and are willing to, pay as their contribution; and (2) the fact that the underlying costs to the service provider of deploying fiber often are substantially the same regardless of whether a 10-25 Mbps connection or 100 Mbps connection is ultimately provided over that fiber. As two projects note, once a fiber connection is in place, HCPs can receive much more bandwidth for a much smaller additional incremental cost.[201] The Arizona Rural Community Health Information Exchange (ARCHIE), for example, states that before the Pilot Program, the undiscounted monthly Internet access bill for seven bonded T-1 lines (approximately 10 Mbps of bandwidth) was almost $10,000.[202] The Pilot funding enabled ARCHIE to purchase a DS-3 connection (approximately 45 Mbps of bandwidth) at $2,000 a month, effectively providing it three times the capacity it previously had. Similarly, participation in the Pilot enabled the Kentucky Behavioral Telehealth Network to pay nearly the same amount ($400-$500 a month) for a thirty-fold increase in bandwidth (through a 45 Mbps connection) as it was paying for a T-1 line.[203] According to USAC, yet another project, through the use of a fiber IRU, is able to provide 1 Gbps symmetrical service to fifty hospitals at an average cost of $640 per month, per hospital, and will have unlimited flexibility in providing for the broadband needs of its members in the future.[204] This project, through an IRU with a different provider, is also providing a 100 Mbps symmetrical service to a separate group of rural HCPs at a cost of $1,300 per month. These rural HCPs previously paid $700 per month for a T-1 (1.544 Mbps) connection.[205]

---

[197] *See supra* Fig. 15 (average Pilot Program support is approximately $993 (3 to less than 6 Mbps), $1,565 (6 to less than 10 Mbps), and $1,497 (10 to less than 25 Mbps); average HCP contribution is approximately $173 (3 to less than 6 Mbps), $302 (6 to less than 10 Mbps), and $291 (10 to less than 25 Mbps)).

[198] Pilot Conference Call Mar. 13 *Ex Parte* Letter (PMHA *et al.*) at 2.

[199] USAC May 30 Data Letter at 4.

[200] *See supra* Fig. 15 (average Pilot Program support is approximately $1,828 for 25 to less than 100 Mbps services, and $1,669 for 100 Mbps or more; average HCP contribution is approximately $329 for 25 to less than 100 Mbps services, and $317 for 100 Mbps or more).

[201] *Id.*

[202] *Id.*

[203] Pilot Conference Call Mar. 16 *Ex Parte* Letter (ARCHIE *et al.*) at 1.

[204] *Id.*

[205] USAC May 30 Data Letter at 3-4.

62. Finally, because a wide variety of HCP types are eligible for support under the Act, different categories of HCPs will have different bandwidth needs and financial resources to pay for those needs. As Figure 16 below shows, hospitals on average tend to pay the most for services, and rural health clinics tend to pay the least.

Figure 16 – Pilot Projects Average Monthly Recurring Cost By HCP Type[206]

Type of HCP	# of HCPs	Average Recurring Cost Per Month		
		Pilot Program Support	HCP Contribution	Total Cost
Rural Health Clinic or Urban Equivalent	392	$1,018	$181	$1,199
Local Health Department or Agency	76	$1,056	$186	$1,242
Community Mental Health Center	272	$1,257	$228	$1,485
Community / Migrant Health Center	281	$1,394	$259	$1,653
Teaching Hospital, Medical School, Post-Secondary Institution	24	$1,467	$259	$1,725
Not-For-Profit Hospital / Dedicated ER of Rural, For-Profit Hospital	500	$1,955	$392	$2,347

IV. IMPROVEMENTS IN QUALITY AND COST OF HEALTH CARE

63. The Pilot Program has helped participating health care providers create local, regional and even state-wide health care networks, resulting in improved quality and lower costs of health care in rural areas. For example, telemedicine is improving health care providers' access to specialists, and allowing rural providers to offer health care to patients that would otherwise have to travel great distances to see medical specialists or forego care entirely. As pointed out by the National Rural Health Resource Center, "telemedicine applications will be crucial in helping to address current and projected shortages in primary care and rural physicians nationwide, as well as shortages of pharmacists in rural areas."[207] The broadband networks created through the Pilot Program also have enabled rural health

---

[206] USAC Aug. 9 Data Letter at App. N.

[207] NRHRC Dec. 27 *Ex Parte* Letter at 2. There are many factors other than the cost or availability of broadband connectivity that affect the pace of adoption of telemedicine. These include lack of reimbursement for services, state licensing requirements, credentialing requirements, lack of technical expertise, and the need for standards. *See, e.g., id.* 2 (noting that the "lack of reimbursement is the biggest obstacle to the deployment of telemedicine services"); Bart M. Demaerschalk, *Telemedicine or Telephone Consultation in Patients with Acute Stroke*, Current Neurology and Neuroscience Reports, Vol. 11: No. 1, 43 (2011) (noting that major barriers to telemedicine adoption include inadequate reimbursement rates, licensing restrictions, lack of reliable internet connectivity, and poor understanding of technology, among others); Rural Maryland Council, *Final Report of the December 2010 Maryland Telehealth and Telemedicine Roundtable* (Jan. 2011), *available at* http://www.rural.state md.us/Roundtables/Telehealth_2010/THTM_Roundtable_FINAL_Jan2011.pdf (last visited June 15, 2012) (concluding that four major barriers to telehealth implementation exist within Maryland: inadequate funding and reimbursement, a lack of state coordination and oversight efforts, broadband limitations, and legal impediments such as licensing); NRHA Dec. 21 *Ex Parte* Letter at 1 ("budget limitations and the shortage of technology personnel" limit adoption of telemedicine in rural areas); NRHRC Dec. 27 *Ex Parte* Letter at 1 and attachments (describing the shortage in health IT workforce in rural areas).

care providers to reduce their often high travel expenses and patient transfer costs, as well as to realize reductions in human resource and administrative expenses. Those networks also have facilitated the sharing of technical and medical expertise and the training of health care personnel in remote areas.[208] Additionally, some Pilot Program health care providers note that telemedicine and telehealth have provided new opportunities to increase revenue. We discuss the impact of the Pilot Program on each of these aspects of health care delivery below.

A.   Telehealth/Telemedicine Applications Enabled by the Pilot Program

64. Pilot projects have been able to deploy a wide range of telehealth and telemedicine applications over their broadband networks. Using these networks, health care providers are able to exchange electronic health records and use other health IT applications; transmit X-rays, MRI, and CT scans and other medical images; and provide distance education, training, and consultation. As discussed below, these applications improve the quality of health care delivered to patients in rural areas, generate savings in the cost of providing this health care, and reduce the time and expense associated with travel to distant locations to receive or provide care.

65. Pilot Projects have reported adoption of a wide variety of telemedicine and telehealth applications, as summarized below in Figure 17. Because many of the Pilot projects are not yet fully implemented, and because not all Pilot projects describe their telemedicine and telehealth activities in their quarterly reports, the figure shows that a relatively small percentage of projects have implemented each type of telehealth application to date. When all the Pilot projects are fully implemented, there is likely to be an even wider adoption of telehealth and telemedicine applications over their networks. The most commonly reported telemedicine applications include tele-psychiatry/tele-psychology, tele-radiology, tele-echocardiology, and tele-stroke. The most commonly reported other telehealth applications include medical training, electronic health records, and tele-pharmacy.

Figure 17 – Telemedicine/Telehealth Applications Reported by Pilot Projects[209]

Telemedicine/Telehealth Application	Count	Percentage of Pilot Projects Using Application
Tele-Psychology/Tele-Psychiatry	9	18%
Continuing medical education	8	16%
Electronic Health Records	7	14%
Tele-Radiology	7	14%
Tele-Echocardiology	6	12%
Tele-Stroke	5	10%
Tele-Pharmacy	4	8%
Tele-ICU	3	6%
Tele-Emergency or Tele-Trauma	3	6%
Tele-Maternal/Fetal Monitoring	3	6%
Tele-Pathology	3	6%
Tele-Infectious Diseases	2	4%
Tele-EEG	1	2%
Tele-Dermatology	1	2%
Other[210]	11	22%

---

[208] See, e.g., NRHRC Ex Parte Letter at 1; USAC Mar. 16 Site Visit Reports at 11 (describing Palmetto State Providers Network's provision of remote training for medical personnel).

[209] Based on staff review of Pilot participant 2011-2012 quarterly reports.

66. Some specific examples of the telehealth and telemedicine applications currently being deployed over Pilot-funded broadband networks include:

- *Palmetto State Providers Network* (PSPN). As of June 2011, over 6,600 tele-psychiatry consults have taken place over PSPN's network, and PSPN conducts 100 tele-OB/GYN, maternal, and fetal care visits per week.[211] Expectant mothers can receive care from fetal medicine specialists, genetic counselors, dietitians and other specialists through the PSPN connection from anywhere in the country.[212]

- *Geisinger Health System* (Geisinger). Geisinger uses its network for numerous telemedicine applications, such as tele-trauma, tele-stroke, tele-echo-cardiology, tele-electroencephalograms (EEG), tele-ICU, tele-psychology, tele-radiology, tele-maternal fetal monitoring and tele-pathology.[213] In 2010, for example, 356 pediatric tele-echo, 432 tele-trauma, and 51 tele-stroke cases were handled through Geisinger's network.[214] The HITECH Act has also led Geisinger to implement health information exchanges (HIEs)[215] over its network.[216]

- *Heartland Unified Broadband Network* (HUBNet). HUBNet provides three examples of improvements facilitated by the Pilot Program. First, following the installation of its HUBNet connection, Horizon Health Care, a consortium of rural clinics in South Dakota, tripled its number of telehealth sessions from ten to thirty sessions per week.[217] Second, HUBNet reports that prior to the Pilot Program, its e-ICU program lacked sufficient bandwidth for two-way video, and patients were reportedly uncomfortable being treated

---

(. . . continued from previous page) ——————————————

[210] Other telehealth applications, as reported by Pilot participants in their quarterly reports, include: orthopedics, ear nose and throat, pediatrician care, general telehealth, neurology, nephrology, diabetes education, and wound care.

[211] USAC Mar. 16 Site Visit Reports at 9; PSPN Mar. 27 *Ex Parte* Letter at 1.

[212] USAC Mar. 16 Site Visit Reports at 10.

[213] *Id.* at 4.

[214] *Id.* at 3.

[215] Health information exchange (HIE) refers to the process of reliable and interoperable electronic health-related information sharing conducted in a manner that protects the confidentiality, privacy, and security of the information. National Alliance for Health Information Technology, *Report to the Office of the National Coordinator for Health Information Technology on Defining Key Health Information Technology Terms* 23 (Apr. 28, 2008), *available at* http://healthit hhs.gov/portal/server.pt/community/healthit hhs gov reports/1239. The HITECH Act provided grants to states and qualified State Designated Entities "to develop and advance mechanisms for information sharing across the health care system." U.S. Department of Health and Human Services, HITECH Priority Grants Program, *available at* http://www hhs.gov/recovery/programs/hitech/stateinfoexch html (last visited June 15, 2012).

[216] USAC Mar. 16 Site Visit Reports at 3. Geisinger is the recipient of a Beacon Communities grant from the Office of the National Coordinator for Health Information Technology of the Department of Health and Human Services to develop a health information exchange over a five county area in northern Pennsylvania. Funded through the HITECH Act, Beacon Recipients were selected "to build and strengthen their HIT infrastructure and exchange capabilities to improve care coordination, increase the quality of care, and slow the growth of health care spending." U.S. Department of Health and Human Services, HHS Awards Affordable Care Act Funds To Improve Quality Of Care And Electronic Reporting Capabilities In Beacon Communities (Sept. 12, 2011), *available at* http://www hhs.gov/news/press/2011pres/09/20110912b.html (last visited June 15, 2012).

[217] USAC Mar. 16 Site Visit Reports at 8.

by a remote physician with an audio-only feed.[218] After implementation of the Pilot Program, HUBNet's e-ICU mobile unit with two-way video service is being used frequently by providers and readily accepted by families.[219] Third, the establishment of tele-pharmacy programs at 27 participating sites has enabled the system to meet Meaningful Use Stage One requirements under the HITECH Act.[220]

- *Oregon Health Network* (OHN). OHN provides tele-stroke, tele-psychiatry, tele-cardiology, tele-dermatology, radiology/PACS/image transfer, continued medical education, and perinatal/Pediatric ICU/Neonatal ICU services over its network. It has 16 members that *provide* telehealth services to 30 members that *receive* telehealth services.[221]

- *Other projects.* Other quantitative measures of telemedicine provided over Pilot-funded networks include: Pathways Community Behavioral Healthcare network (1,000 psychiatric telehealth services per month);[222] Missouri Telehealth Network (4,000 clinical telehealth encounters across 30 medical specialties in 2010);[223] and Southwest Alabama Mental Health Consortium (508 hours of service to 714 individuals located in rural Alabama between August 2011 and January 2012).[224]

- *Health Information Exchanges.* Other projects have also begun developing HIEs over their Pilot-funded networks. The Louisiana Department of Health and Hospitals (LA DHH) Pilot Project, in partnership with the Louisiana Health Care Quality Forum, is currently in the process of developing an HIE.[225] Likewise, the Oregon Health Network plans to serve as the "State's identified HIE broadband infrastructure 'highway,'" to support the exchange of electronic health care records across the state.[226] The North Carolina Telehealth Network also states that a statewide Health Information Exchange is under development in North Carolina, and HCPs will connect to it through PSPN when it becomes operational.[227] The Pennsylvania Mountains Healthcare Resource Development

---

[218] *Id.*

[219] *Id.*

[220] *Id.* at 6-7.

[221] OHN Feb. 28 *Ex Parte* Letter at 3. A PACS is a "picture archiving and communication system," which is an electronic information system for acquiring, sorting, displaying, and storing medical images. *See Picture Archiving and Communications Systems*, AM. MED. ASS'N, http://www.ama-assn.org/ama/pub/physician-resources/health-information-technology/health-it-basics/pacs.page (last visited Aug. 8, 2012).

[222] Quarterly Report of Pathways Community Behavioral Healthcare Quarterly Report, WC Docket No. 02-60, at 14 (filed Jan. 30, 2012).

[223] Quarterly Report of Missouri Telehealth Network, WC Docket No. 02-60, at 5 (filed Jan. 31, 2012).

[224] Quarterly Report of Southwest Alabama Mental Health Consortium, WC Docket No. 02-60, at 15 (filed Jan. 30, 2012). With the availability of video-conferencing equipment, Southwest Alabama Mental Health Consortium notes that it provided psychiatric services to 575 clients in rural Alabama during the same time period. *Id.*

[225] Quarterly Report of Louisiana Department of Health and Hospitals, WC Docket No. 02-60, at 4 (filed Oct. 28, 2011).

[226] Quarterly Report of Oregon Health Network, WC Docket No. 02-60, at 11 (filed Jan. 31, 2012).

[227] USAC Apr. 27 Site Visit Reports at 2.

project reports that all its hospitals will be connecting to a local area and/or statewide health information exchange.[228]

B.   Improved Quality and Efficiency of Health Care Delivery

67. Pilot Projects indicate that telemedicine applications provide increased access to specialty services and emergency care, no matter where a patient may be located. This allows for better, faster treatment for patients.[229] One Pilot project reports that patients and families state that they can now get care in the local, rural hospital that is comparable to the level in the closest urban hospital.[230] Telemedicine can also shorten the length of a patient's stay in the hospital. For example:

- *Tele-stroke.* Geisinger states that its network provides tele-stroke services to neurology consults for patients "within minutes, as opposed to hours."[231] Bacon County Hospital in southeastern Georgia reported an instance when a young woman having a stroke had her life saved because the local physicians were able to use their telemedicine connection to a specialist in Savannah, and as a result were able to administer the clot-busting drug TPA.[232]

- *Tele-psychiatry.* An example of cost savings from telemedicine is the use of tele-psychiatry in the emergency room setting. Rural hospitals might have no choice but to admit a patient presenting psychiatric symptoms while waiting for a psychiatrist to visit in person. A remote video consult with a psychiatrist could enable a rural hospital to diagnose, treat, and discharge the patient rather than admitting the patient for days without treatment. The Palmetto State Providers Network (PSPN) states that prior to the adoption of its tele-psychiatry program, patients would wait days for a psychiatric consult, during which time they would be held in the rural hospital's emergency department. After implementation, however, psychiatric consults are generally available "at any time, with minimal wait."[233] PSPN also notes that all four metropolitan hospitals serving South Carolina now have access to all patient psychiatry records via Electronic

---

[228] USAC Mar. 16 Site Visit Reports at 15.

[229] *See, e.g.,* USAC Mar. 16 Site Visit Reports at 6 (benefits of E-emergency connection includes helping rural medical professionals build relationships with urban counterparts; allowing rural doctor and nurses to focus entirely on patient care, because urban staff assist in coordinating patient transport when needed; helping urban site to provide better care to patients when they have to be transported because the patient's condition has already been assessed remotely; and allowing urban site to make arrangements in advance of a patient's arrival where that patient needs to see a specialist); NRHRC Dec. 27 *Ex Parte* Letter at 2 (stating that telemedicine applications will be crucial to addressing current and projected shortages in primary care and rural physicians nationwide, and that telehealth applications will become increasingly useful and necessary for delivering primary care in rural communities); ONC Jan. 6 *Ex Parte* Letter at 1 (noting research that suggests that only roughly 30 percent of visits require the physical presence of a doctor, and that the medical appropriateness of remote visits is becoming well-established).

[230] *See, e.g.,* USAC Mar. 16 Site Visit Reports at 8.

[231] *Id.* at 3.

[232] USAC Apr. 27 Site Visit Reports at 4. *See also* ONC Jan. 17 *Ex Parte* Letter at 2 (explaining that when the emergency room of a rural hospital is able to quickly transmit a CT scan of a patient's head to a neurologist in an urban hospital, the rural hospital can prevent permanent stroke damage by administering preventative medicine in a timely fashion, but where only a T-1 connection is available, transmission of the CT scan could take 25 minutes, and the delay could have serious consequences for the patient).

[233] USAC Mar. 16 Site Visit Reports at 9.

Medical Records (EMRs) over the PSPN, which has greatly enhanced the urban centers' ability to provide treatment.[234]

- *Tele-OB/GYN.* Prior to the adoption of tele-OB/GYN services through the PSPN network, expectant mothers in some parts of South Carolina would have to travel up to 168 miles to see a doctor, according to a PSPN physician.[235] PSPN also notes that patient visit no-show rates are directly proportional to the price of gasoline and the distance to see a physician.[236] Thus, telemedicine means more high-risk expectant mothers in rural areas are receiving care. Before the tele-OB/GYN program, a PSPN physician would spend six hours a day driving to rural South Carolina to see each patient for only three minutes.[237] Now, through the use of telemedicine, the same physician is now able to utilize the entire working day and spends an average of thirty minutes with each one.[238]

- *Tele-radiology.* The enhanced broadband capabilities at Punxsutawney Hospital, a Pennsylvania Mountains Healthcare Alliance (PMHA) participant, have reduced the turnaround time on X-ray readings from 20 minutes to 7 minutes, allowing for more timely clinical interventions where needed.[239] The network has also eliminated the need to manually create and deliver mammography DVDs at another PMHA hospital, reducing what was once an "inordinate amount" of clinical time to two to three minutes.[240]

- *Electronic Intensive Care (e-ICU).* HUBNet states that its e-ICU program, which allows physicians to monitor vitals, pharmacy orders, and test results, has significantly reduced the number of days, on average, that a patient stays in the intensive care unit.[241]

- *Public Health Monitoring.* The North Carolina Telehealth Network, which focuses on local public health as well as general acute care medicine, has connected public health departments across North Carolina that are using the bandwidth for communicable disease tracking, syndromic surveillance, and environmental health reporting. Communicable disease tracking has allowed the turnaround time on a suspected outbreak to go from 5 to 10 days to 24 to 48 hours.[242]

- *Electronic Health Records.* The Sanford Health Collaboration and Communication Channel notes that the Pilot Program allowed it to upgrade from T-1 connections to Ethernet services, which then enabled the project to roll out EHRs. Having complete EHRs enables this hospital, which has patients coming from as far as 150 miles away from a number of entry points, to treat patients more efficiently and effectively.

---

[234] *Id.*

[235] *Id.* at 10.

[236] *Id.*

[237] *Id.*

[238] *Id.*

[239] *Id.* at 15.

[240] *Id.*

[241] *Id.* at 7.

[242] USAC Apr. 27 Site Visit Reports at 2.

Furthermore, as patients move from specialty to specialty, the patient outcomes are better because all the patient information is centrally captured.[243]

68. An important benefit of the Pilot Program is that increases in bandwidth can improve the quality of telemedicine encounters even where telemedicine programs already exist, which in turn improves the quality of care and staff and patient acceptance of telemedicine. For example, the Jefferson County Hospital in Iowa had Internet VPN connections and residential grade broadband, from multiple service providers, before its Pilot-funded connection. Over the pre-Pilot connection, tele-radiology services took a minimum of 30 to 40 minutes to send images for reading. The time to send images caused significant delay in providing patient services (patient waits were 3-4 hours in length). This hospital now receives a 30 Mbps connection through the Iowa Rural Health Telecommunications Program (IRHTP) Pilot project network, which allows transmission of high-resolution images within 60 seconds (comparable to service in urban areas). Patient wait time is now only 30 minutes, and the hospital reports that the number of misdiagnoses is down dramatically.[244]

69. Another example of the benefits of increased bandwidth is HUBNet's E-emergency telemedicine program. Prior to the Pilot Program, the audio and video components of this program were frequently not synchronized, especially if more than one person was in the room. At times, the E-emergency program had to be turned off and rebooted for the connection to work properly. HUBNet reports that the increased bandwidth has dramatically improved the ability to provide quality care to patients through the telemedicine program.[245]

70. USAC's Pilot project site visit reports indicate that once telemedicine programs are implemented and operational, nearly all physicians and patients report positive, high levels of acceptance of telemedicine applications. One HUBNet hospital administrator reported that its staff is now "heavily dependent on the connection" and that "increased bandwidth speed is the single best process change they have done."[246] Another HUBNet hospital reports that tele-consult visits are "so popular within the community that the patients are now the ones asking for tele-consults."[247] Many Pilot projects report enhancement of physician satisfaction and collegial support due to telemedicine applications provided over the Pilot-funded broadband networks.[248] Physicians appreciate the ability to consult with other colleagues, especially in remote areas. Geisinger notes that telemedicine has enhanced "physician recruitment, retention, satisfaction, and collegial support," noting that applications such as e-ICU allow physicians to "practice in a rural setting knowing that specialized help [is] only seconds away."[249] Telemedicine also enables Pilot participants such as Northwest Alabama Mental Health Center to "attract qualified health professionals due to [their] new tele-psychiatry services which reduces travel

---

[243] Pilot Conference Call Mar. 26 *Ex Parte* Letter (WNYRAHEC *et al.*) at 1-2. *See also* USAC Mar. 16 Site Visit Reports at 14 (stating that Henry County Health Center, part of the IRHTP, was one of the first HCPs in the country to reach stage one meaningful use requirements, and that the health center uses the broadband connection for all of its EMRs).

[244] USAC Mar. 16 Site Visit Reports at 13-14.

[245] *Id.* at 5.

[246] *Id.* at 5, 8.

[247] *Id.* at 8.

[248] *See, e.g.,* USAC Mar. 16 Site Visit Reports at 3, 4, 8, 11, 14, 15; USAC Apr. 27 Site Visit Reports at 2-3 .

[249] USAC Mar. 16 Site Visit Reports at 3.

time and increases the number of patient visits that can be made."[250] One Pilot project cites a study showing that recruitment and retention of doctors and health professionals in rural areas can be positively impacted by the use of telehealth.[251]

71. Finally, Pilot networks also offer training opportunities for medical personnel in rural areas. For example, PSPN states that 25 continuing education courses were offered to 457 health care providers within a 7-month period in 2011, and physician's assistant students on rotation throughout the PSPN sites were trained remotely during July and August 2011.[252]

C. Cost Savings from Telemedicine/Telehealth Applications

1. Reduced Transfer and Travel Costs

72. Telemedicine provides patients in rural areas the opportunity to be diagnosed and/or treated in their own communities, and can provide significant savings by reducing patient transfer or physician, patient, and/or family travel costs. As one project states, linking to urban centers and using telemedicine "bends the cost curve."[253] Overall, ten Pilot participants report that telemedicine currently provides, or in the future would likely provide, savings in the form of reduced travel costs.[254] Examples of savings in transfer and/or travel costs facilitated by the Pilot Program include the following:

- Heartland Unified Broadband Network (HUBNet) estimates that over a thirty-month period, eight hospitals in its network have saved a total of $1.2 million in transfer expenses following the implementation of e-ICU services.[255] This estimate did not include the additional savings due to avoiding provision of care at the urban site, nor did it take into account the revenue that otherwise would have been lost by the rural site, or the savings by patients' families, who avoided travel to urban locations.[256] Other

---

[250] Quarterly Report of Northwest Alabama Mental Health Center, WC Docket No. 02-60, at 7 (filed July 29, 2011); *see also* USAC Apr. 27 Site Visit Reports at 3 (stating that telemedicine technology has had a positive impact on Bacon County Hospital's ability to recruit and retain physicians).

[251] Quarterly Report of Missouri Telehealth Network, WC Docket No. 02-60, at 6 (filed Apr. 30, 2012) (citing Duplantie, J., Gagnon, M., Fortin, J., & Landry, R. (2007), Telehealth and the recruitment and retention of physicians in rural and remote regions: a Delphi study, Canadian Journal Of Rural Medicine, 12(1), 30-36).

[252] USAC Mar. 16 Site Visit Reports at 11.

[253] Pilot Conference Call Mar. 26 *Ex Parte* Letter (WNYRAHEC *et al.*) at 2-3.

[254] Quarterly Report of Communicare, WC Docket No. 02-60, at 5 (filed Jan. 30, 2012); Quarterly Report of Heartland Unified Broadband Network, WC Docket No. 02-60, at 56 (filed Jan. 30, 2012); Quarterly Report of Missouri Telehealth Network, WC Docket No. 02-60, at 5 (filed Jan. 31, 2012); Quarterly Report of Northwest Alabama Mental Health Center, WC Docket No. 02-60, at 6 (filed July 29, 2011); Quarterly Report of Pathways Community Behavioral Healthcare, WC Docket No. 02-60, at 14 (filed Jan. 30, 2012); Quarterly Report of Southwest Alabama Mental Health Consortium, WC Docket No. 02-60, at 9 (filed Jan. 30, 2012); Quarterly Report of Southwest Telehealth Access Grid, WC Docket No. 02-60, at 14 (filed Jan. 27, 2012); USAC Mar. 16 Site Visit Reports at 3 n.1 (regarding Geisinger Health System); USAC Mar. 16 Site Visit Reports at 11 (regarding Palmetto State Providers Network); OHN Feb. 28 *Ex Parte* Letter at 4 (stating that one hour of air transfer costs approximately $24,000).

[255] USAC Mar. 16 Site Visit Reports at 7.

[256] *Id.*

participants, such as Geisinger and the Missouri Telehealth Network (MTN), also cite reduced transfer costs as tangible benefits from telemedicine applications.[257]

- HUBNet and MTN also cite to reduced patient travel as a sizable cost-saving measure brought about by an increase in telemedicine and telehealth applications. MTN reports that in 2009, its patients avoided 1,700 round trips from rural areas of Missouri to specialist clinics in Columbia and Kirksville, saving 538,000 miles of travel and over $293,000 in fuel costs alone.[258] HUBNet relies on a study at Avera Milbank Hospital (a Critical Access Hospital) demonstrating that, over the course of a year, telemedicine allowed 67 patients to stay in their local community to receive treatment instead of traveling 152 miles away to Sioux Falls.[259]

2.   Reduced Operating Costs and Increased Revenue Opportunities

73. Telemedicine and telehealth can also demonstrably reduce providers' operating costs by lowering the cost of delivering health care, minimizing human resource expenses, and reducing administrative costs.[260] The National Rural Health Resource Center explains that health IT can help rural hospitals to provide care for rural residents in their communities for less cost, and notes that most overtreatment, which accounts for one-third of national spending on health care, takes place in major heath care centers rather than small rural hospitals.[261] Several Pilot Program participants report lower costs as a result of the program. For example:

- PSPN reports that Emergency Department psychiatry treatment costs dropped from $2,500 to $400 per patient, per day as a result of its tele-psychiatry program.[262] As a result, PSPN has realized $18 million dollars in Medicaid savings.[263] Prior to the adoption of its tele-psychiatry program, PSPN notes that patients could wait days for a psychiatric consult, during which time the patient would be held in the rural hospital's

---

[257] Geisinger reports that its e-ICU program at Lewistown and Evangelical Hospital allows for reduced travel expenses by avoiding $10,000 helicopter and two-to-three-hour ground transports to locations that provide more specialized care. *See* USAC Mar. 16 Site Visit Reports at 3, n.1. MTN estimates that each transport from the Marshall Habilitation Center (MHC), located in Marshall, Missouri, to the University of Missouri (UM), located in Columbia, Missouri, costs MHC more than $500 per patient. Quarterly Report of Missouri Telehealth Network, WC Docket No. 02-60, at 6 (filed Jan. 31, 2012).

[258] MTN notes that the average savings per trip was $175.00. *Id.*

[259] Quarterly Report of Missouri Telehealth Network, WC Docket No. 02-60, at 6 (filed Jan. 31, 2012).

[260] *See, e.g.,* Quarterly Report of Southwest Telehealth Access Grid, WC Docket No. 02-60, at 14 (filed Jan. 27, 2012) (stating that it anticipates reduced costs as result of "improved sharing of resources"); Quarterly Report of Southwest Alabama Mental Health Consortium, WC Docket No. 02-60, at 10 (filed Jan. 27, 2012) (stating that the use of electronic health records will bring "increased staff productivity"); Quarterly Report of Tennessee Telehealth Network, WC Docket No. 02-60, at 11 (filed Jan. 31, 2012) (stating that it anticipates that increased savings will be realized from administrative efficiencies, including the sharing of practice management, electronic health records, and participating in a health information exchange across the network).

[261] NRHRC Dec. 27 *Ex Parte* Letter at 2.

[262] USAC Mar. 16 Site Visit Reports at 10.

[263] PSPN Feb. 23 *Ex Parte* Letter at 1. *See also* PSPN Mar. 27 *Ex Parte* Letter at 1.

emergency department.[264] After implementation, however, fewer resources were devoted to patients waiting for evaluations.[265]

- The Adirondack Champlain Telemedicine Information Network (ACTION) anticipates $9 million in future operating cost savings as a direct result of the provision of tele-cardiology, tele-trauma, tele-mental health, tele-neurology, and tele-respiratory services.[266]

- One PMHRD hospital states that the transmission of clinical and financial information over their network has reduced employee turnover because employees are now able to do transcription work from home.[267] Since the network was implemented, it notes that the turnover rate for transcriptionists dropped from fifty to zero percent, saving the hospital approximately $20,000 per full time employee.[268] PMHRD also states that the network has enabled the development of a revenue cycle management program that has the potential to increase an HCP's bottom line by 2-3 percent, as well as reduced operating costs.[269]

- The Northwest Alabama Mental Health Center reported that it foresees savings as a result of "reduced intercompany long distance phone calls, number of telephone lines, [and] travel incurred by staff psychiatrists."[270]

- The Satilla Regional Medical Center in Georgia, through its e-ICU program, has been able to reduce patient lengths of stay and ventilator treatment days with no denigration of care and with substantial cost savings to the Medical Center.[271]

74. Telemedicine applications have also created opportunities for increased revenue streams for rural Pilot participants. By keeping patients in rural hospitals, and by continuing to serve patients in rural clinics, telemedicine can provide rural HCPs with opportunities to retain or increase their revenues.[272] Most rural HCPs operate on a very thin margin, and many operate at a loss.[273] For rural HCPs, broadband connections mean they can use telemedicine to retain patients and consult with specialists remotely, "Which is better for patients and helps rural hospitals financially."[274] For example,

---

[264] USAC Mar. 16 Site Visit Reports at 10.

[265] *Id.*

[266] Quarterly Report of Adirondack Champlain Telemedicine Information Network, WC Docket No. 02-60, at 5 (filed Jan. 20, 2012).

[267] USAC Mar. 16 Site Visit Reports at 15.

[268] *Id.*

[269] *Id.*

[270] Quarterly Report of Northwest Alabama Mental Health Center, WC Docket No. 02-60, at 6 (filed July 29, 2011).

[271] USAC Apr. 27 Site Visit Reports at 3.

[272] ORHP Apr. 10 *Ex Parte* Letter at 2. *See also* NRHRC Dec. 27 *Ex Parte* Letter at 2 ("Having more patients receive care locally…helps rural hospitals to be successful."); USAC Mar. 16 Site Visit Reports at 2.

[273] *See* NRHA Dec. 21 *Ex Parte* Letter at 1; NRHRC Dec. 27 *Ex Parte* Letter at 2 (many critical access hospitals and other small rural hospitals "are experiencing negative margins and facing increasing difficulties in accessing capital"). *See also* USAC Mar. 16 Site Visit Reports at 14 (Jefferson County Hospital in Iowa reports that it can keep more patients in the local hospital because of the quick send and read of the radiology scans).

[274] *See* Pilot Conference Call Mar. 16 *Ex Parte* Letter at 1-2 (ARCHIE *et al.*) at 1-2. *See generally* NRHRC Dec. 27 *Ex Parte* Letter at 2 (discussing how telemedicine allows rural hospitals to treat patients locally); *see also* ORHP

(continued . . .)

in the HUBNet Avera Milbank Hospital study, the use of telemedicine enabled a rural critical access hospital to provide $24,456 in services locally that would otherwise have been provided elsewhere, including specialist order services such as bone scans, ultrasounds, x-rays, CT studies, and various lab tests.[275] PMHA states that its network has enabled the development of a revenue cycle management program with the potential to increase a rural provider's revenue stream by two to three percent, as well as reduce operating costs.[276] Finally, broadband connections can be used to address shortages of health IT personnel in rural areas by facilitating training via video conference.[277]

75. In addition to those projects that have already started to realize increased revenues as a result of their broadband networks, Pilot projects whose networks are not yet operational anticipate that telemedicine applications will increase their revenue. The North Country Telemedicine Project (NCTP) predicts that telemedicine capabilities will enhance local inpatient hospital revenue by nearly $4.1 million due to increased retention of patients across five specialties – general surgery, cardiology, gastroenterology, oncology, and pulmonology.[278] Currently, patients from these specialties represent more than 20 percent of cases that are transferred from local NCTP health care centers to urban hospitals.[279] Likewise, St. Joseph's Hospital projects that initial telehealth services for ER, ICU and behavioral health will generate $25,000 in revenue each year.[280] In total, 15 Pilot sites noted in their quarterly reports that they plan to rely on revenue from telemedicine services to offset future network costs, with many emphasizing tele-behavioral health services in particular, due to Medicare and Medicaid reimbursement polices.[281] The Kentucky Behavioral Telehealth Network Sustainability Report

(. . . continued from previous page) ————————————————————————

Apr. 10 *Ex Parte* Letter at 2 (explaining that rural hospitals are reimbursed a facility fee when they seek service from a physician at an urban location *via* telemedicine).

[275] Quarterly Report of Heartland Unified Broadband Network, WC Docket No. 02-60, at 56 (filed Jan. 30, 2012).

[276] USAC Mar. 16 Site Visit Reports at 15.

[277] *See, e.g.,* NRHRC Dec. 27 *Ex Parte* Letter at 1 (vendors are conducting much of the training for implementation of electronic health record systems via video conference, due to the shortage in health IT workforce).

[278] Quarterly Report of North Country Telemedicine Project, WC Docket No. 02-60, at 29 (filed Jan. 30, 2012).

[279] *Id.*

[280] Quarterly Report of St. Joseph Hospital, WC Docket No. 02-60, at 8 (filed Jan. 20, 2012).

[281] Quarterly Report of Adirondack Champlain Telemedicine Information Network, WC Docket No. 02-60, at 18 (filed Jan. 20, 2012); Quarterly Report of Frontier Access to Rural Healthcare in Montana, WC Docket No. 02-60, at 11 (filed Jan. 12, 2012); Quarterly Report of Geisinger Health System, WC Docket No. 02-60, at 3 (filed Jan. 25, 2012); Quarterly Report of Heartland Unified Broadband Network, WC Docket No. 02-60, at 56 (filed Jan. 30, 2012); Quarterly Report of Kentucky Behavioral Telehealth Network, WC Docket No. 02-60, at 29 (filed Jan. 30, 2012); Quarterly Report of North Country Telemedicine Project, WC Docket No. 02-60, at 27 (filed Jan. 30, 2012); Quarterly Report of Northeast HealthNet, WC Docket No. 02-60, at 12 (filed Dec. 31, 2011); Quarterly Report of Northwest Alabama Mental Health Center, WC Docket No. 02-60, at 6 (filed July 29, 2011); Quarterly Report of Northwestern Pennsylvania Telemedicine Initiative, WC Docket No. 02-60, at 6, 9 (filed Jan. 25, 2012); Quarterly Report of Pacific Broadband Telehealth Demonstration Project, WC Docket No. 02-60, at 10 (filed Oct. 25, 2011); Quarterly Report of Pathways Community Behavioral Healthcare, WC Docket No. 02-60, at 14 (filed Jan. 30, 2012); Quarterly Report of Pennsylvania Mountains Healthcare Alliance, WC Docket No. 02-60, at 14 (filed Feb. 6, 2012); Quarterly Report of Southwest Telehealth Access Grid, WC Docket No. 02-60, at 13 (filed Jan. 27, 2012); Quarterly Report of St. Joseph's Hospital, WC Docket No. 02-60, at 8 (filed Jan. 20, 2012); Quarterly Report of Tennessee Telehealth Network, WC Docket No. 02-60, at 11 (filed Jan. 31, 2012); *see also* Centers for Medicare and Medicaid Services, *Rural Health Fact Sheet Series: Telehealth Services* (February 2012), http://www.cms.gov/Outreach-and-Education/Medicare-Learning-Network-MLN/MLNProducts/downloads/TelehealthSrvcsfctsht.pdf; Center for Telehealth e-Health Law, *50 State Survey on Medicaid Telehealth and Telehomecare Policies (Parts 1-3)* (February 2011), *available at* http://ctel.org/expertise/reimbursement/medicaid-reimbursement/.

specifically noted that Kentucky state law mandates Medicaid reimbursement of tele-behavioral health services at the same rate as face-to-face services.[282] Likewise, the Northwest Alabama Mental Health Center and Pathways Community Behavioral Healthcare notes that it anticipates opportunities for increased psychiatric billing.[283] Other alternative revenue streams reported by Pilot participants also include marketing agreements with Health IT product vendors[284] and leasing of excess capacity on constructed fiber lines.[285]

V.   KEY OBSERVATIONS

76. As part of this evaluation, Commission staff sought input from Pilot Program participants and from USAC about their experiences with the Pilot Program. According to many Pilot participants, the key features of the Pilot Program were the consortium approach, the inclusion of urban providers, the broad definition of eligible expenses, the use of multi-year commitments (*e.g.*, IRUs and long-term prepaid leases), the use of a flat-rate discount approach, and the size of the discount. In its role as Administrator, USAC also provided valuable insights about its experience with the Pilot Program and its benefits.[286] Some of the projects also identified several challenges, including the exclusion of administrative expenses and the difficulty of predicting the long-term sustainability of the Pilot projects. We discuss various key observations below.

A.   Use of Consortia

77. To facilitate the funding of broadband health care provider networks, the Commission required HCPs to apply to the Pilot Program as consortia.[287] The consortium application approach proved to have many benefits both for the Pilot projects and for USAC as the program administrator. It has simplified the application process for HCPs and USAC, resulted in significant cost savings for participants, and contributed to administrative efficiencies.[288] As a representative of the National Rural Health Association put it, "permitting providers to apply for support as part of a consortium application would be of great help, especially for smaller providers such as rural health clinics, which have few administrative resources and for whom turn over in administrative personnel can pose a problem."[289]

78. *Simplicity of Application Process.* Applying as a consortium is simpler, cheaper, and more efficient for the health care providers than the Primary Program application process, which requires a separate application for each HCP each year.[290] In the Pilot Program, projects are required to file just a

---

[282] Quarterly Report of Kentucky Behavioral Telehealth Network, WC Docket No. 02-60, at 29 (filed Jan. 27, 2012).

[283] Quarterly Report of Northwest Alabama Mental Health Center, WC Docket No. 02-60, at 6 (filed July 29, 2011).

[284] Quarterly Report of Colorado Health Care Connections, WC Docket No. 02-60, at 11 (filed Jan. 27, 2012); Quarterly Report of Rocky Mountain Health Net, WC Docket No. 02-60, at 10 (filed Jan. 27, 2012).

[285] Quarterly Report of Erlanger, WC Docket No. 02-60, at 13 (filed Jan. 30, 2012); Quarterly Report of Rural Nebraska Healthcare Network, WC Docket No. 02-60, at 8 (filed Jan. 26, 2012); Quarterly Report of Health Information Exchange of Montana, WC Docket No. 02-60, at 10 (filed Jan. 24, 2012).

[286] *See, e.g.,* USAC Observations Letter; USAC Mar. 16 and Apr. 27 Site Visit Reports; USAC Needs Assessment.

[287] *2006 Pilot Program Order,* 21 FCC Rcd at 11111-12, 11116-17, paras. 1, 3, 16-17.

[288] *See generally* USAC Observations Letter at 2-4.

[289] NRHA Dec. 21 *Ex Parte* Letter at 1; *see also* NRHRC Dec. 27 *Ex Parte* Letter at 2.

[290] *See generally* USAC Observations Letter at 2-3; Pilot Conference Call Mar. 26 *Ex Parte* Letter (WNYRAHEC *et al.*) at 4 (noting view of six Pilot projects that the consortium-based approach in the Pilot Program is much easier than the process in the Primary Program).

single Form 465 and 466 that includes information on the individual HCP sites in their network.[291] Some Pilot projects have hundreds of sites, but still file only one application. In contrast, even though the Primary Program permits consortium applications, that program requires a separate application for each consortium-member HCP site, and requires HCPs to file those applications annually.[292] For rural HCPs considering participation in the Primary Program, the administrative cost of filing a separate application sometimes can outweigh the benefit of the anticipated discount.[293] Also, smaller HCPs often lack the administrative resources and technical expertise to participate.[294] High levels of administrative staff turnover at rural HCPs can present a further challenge, especially if applications have to be resubmitted annually.[295]

79. As noted below, the use of a flat-rate discount applicable to all eligible expenses in the Pilot Program is administratively simpler for applicants and for USAC, and makes it easier to pursue consortium applications with many HCP sites. The flat discount also makes it easier for each HCP to determine the level of funding it would receive and thus to evaluate whether it is worth participating in the program, compared with determining the urban/rural discount that would be available in the Primary Program.[296] Some HCPs also recognize that the ability to bill service providers as a consortium in the Pilot Program is helpful.[297]

80. *Advantages for USAC Application Review Process.* The use of consortium applications in the Pilot Program has also enabled USAC to review applications with many individual sites at once and to make determinations regarding those applications in a more efficient, consolidated fashion.[298] For example, because they operate as consortia, Pilot projects are required to obtain Letters of Agency (LOA) from participating HCPs in their networks, which has helped USAC determine participant eligibility.[299] Additionally, because consortium applicants have a centralized approach to the application and network design process, they are able to respond more efficiently to USAC throughout the application process.[300] Finally, the consortium application process provides USAC the ability to

---

[291] *2007 Pilot Program Selection Order*, 22 FCC Rcd at 20405, 20407, paras. 86, 89.

[292] *See* 47 C.F.R. §§ 54.603(b), 54.623(d); USAC Observations Letter at 2.

[293] *See* NRHA Dec. 21 *Ex Parte* Letter at 1 (noting that some health care providers do not complete the application process because of uncertainty about how much of a discount they will receive).

[294] *See id.* at 1; Pilot Conference Call Mar. 13 *Ex Parte* Letter (PMHA *et al.)* at 3 (noting view of five Pilot projects that a reformed RHC program should provide opportunities for networks to file as consortia, which takes the administrative burden off of small HCPs that do not have the time or personnel to apply for funds through the RHC program, and that the ability to bill service providers as a consortium in the Pilot Program was very helpful); PSPN Feb. 23 *Ex Parte* Letter at 2 (stating individual health care providers often do not have the capacity to negotiate RHC processes and that the ability to bill as a consortium is more efficient than requiring hundreds of members to submit invoices each month); NCTN Apr. 9 *Ex Parte* Letter at 2 (stating that the NCTN's formation of a consortium has been very successful, by lowering administrative costs, improving appropriate uptake of services, improving completion, improving operations, and providing a nexus for supporting broadband-related health projects in North Carolina; and strongly encouraging the Commission to support such consortia in a reformed RHC program).

[295] *See* NRHA Dec. 21 *Ex Parte* Letter at 1; NRHRC Dec. 27 *Ex Parte* Letter at 2.

[296] *See infra* Section V.H.

[297] Pilot Conference Call Mar. 13 *Ex Parte* Letter (PMHA *et al.*) at 3; PSPN Feb. 23 *Ex Parte* Letter at 2.

[298] USAC Observations Letter at 2-4.

[299] *Id.* at 3.

[300] *See id.* at 2-4.

substitute HCPs and services in the networks more efficiently. USAC explains that because HCP circuits in the Pilot Program are funded at the consortium level, it can substitute or modify the site or service without modifying the actual commitment level.[301] This is more efficient than the Primary Program, in which any modification of funding requires a new application and a new funding commitment letter for each HCP impacted.[302]

81. *Lower Rates, Higher Bandwidth, and Better Service Quality.* The consortium bulk buying capability of multiple HCPs, combined with the RFP and competitive bidding process, has enabled many Pilot projects to obtain lower rates for services and to realize other purchasing efficiencies.[303] Applicants for rural health care support must select the most cost effective vendor through a competitive bidding process. In the Primary Program, USAC estimates that bids are received for services representing only 16 percent of funding requests; the remainder do not receive competitive bids after posting for such bids.[304] The consortium approach in the Pilot Program, however, appears to have made the competitive bidding process more fruitful, as 24 projects had 6 or more vendors bid on some component of the project, and 14 had more than ten vendors bid.[305] Furthermore, all but 3 projects had more than a single vendor bid.[306] Through this process, over 120 vendors have been selected to provide services to the Pilot Projects. A list of winning vendors is attached as Appendix D and includes large communications providers; small, rural local exchange providers; cable operators; municipal electric utilities; construction companies; and systems integrators.

82. Some of the communications service providers bidding on the RFPs also may be more willing to offer Pilot projects larger discounts because the Pilot projects have multiple sites and present a more appealing commercial proposition to the service providers.[307] Also, when one or more large health care providers is a part of the project (typically those providers are located in urban areas), vendors may be more interested in bidding on the projects and in offering competitive rates to all the sites, as a way to attract the business of the larger HCPs.[308] In addition, because a single RFP includes all HCP sites (both those that have broadband available to them and those that do not), vendors often must bid on providing

---

[301] *Id.* at 3-4.

[302] *Id.* at 4.

[303] Colorado Telehealth Network and others note that operating as consortia has provided them greater purchasing (*i.e.* bulk-buying) power, which has allowed them to negotiate lower pricing with their service provider. Colorado Feb. 28 *Ex Parte* Letter at 1 (stating that financial benefits have accrued to member HCPs from the joint purchasing power that led to a cost-effective contract with the communications service provider); *see also* OHN Feb. 28 *Ex Parte* Letter at 1 (stating that OHN's multi-vendor leased line network framework helped utilize the existing state fiber infrastructure while creating the highest level of competition possible, allowing smaller local service providers to compete directly and fairly with larger providers, which subsequently resulted in OHN's members receiving the most competitive bids (reduced costs) possible); Pilot Conference Call Mar. 13 *Ex Parte* Letter (PMHA *et al.*) at 2 (stating that the benefits of pilot funding include the ability to obtain Internet services as a group); Pilot Conference Call Mar. 26 *Ex Parte* Letter (WNYRAHEC *et al.*) at 2 (WNYRAHEC stating that it has experienced a great deal of cost savings from being on a shared network).

[304] USAC May 30 Data Letter at 2. If no bids are received in response to a Form 465 request for services, a health care provider may then contact its local service provider and enter into a contract. *Id.* at 1.

[305] USAC May 30 Data Letter at 2.

[306] *Id.*

[307] *See* USAC Aug. 2 Data Letter at 4; *see also* USAC Observations Letter at 1-2 (use of centralized contracting and invoicing; use of Master Services Agreements).

[308] *See, e.g.,* UVA June 8 *Ex Parte* Letter at 2.

broadband connections to sites where broadband might not already be available.[309] For the majority of Pilot projects, the competitive bidding process itself also has been successful in attracting multiple bids from a range of different service providers.[310]

83. In addition to attracting lower rates, the consortium-based competitive bidding process has produced other purchasing efficiencies. The project-wide RFP and competitive bidding process often requires vendors to work with a number of underlying communications service providers, and to assemble offerings from a number of sources, in order to provide service as requested in the RFP.[311] This reduces the burden on Pilot projects, as they do not have to negotiate and contract with a number of different service providers to create their networks.[312] Also, vendors bidding on the projects are responsible for ensuring that necessary service quality, reliability, and interoperability requirements specified in the RFP are fulfilled.[313] As a result, bulk buying and competitive bidding, and the consortium contract negotiations, appear to enhance the ability of rural HCPs to obtain not just higher bandwidth connections than otherwise, but also to secure better service quality and reliability guarantees from service providers.[314] Finally, the provision of multi-year funding under the Pilot Program (and the permissibility of multi-year contracts and prepaid leases) may encourage term discounts and may produce lower rates from vendors.[315]

84. *Cost Savings through Centralization and Sharing of Administrative Expenses.* Under the consortium approach, the expenses associated with planning the network, applying for funding, issuing RFPs, contracting with service providers, and invoicing are shared among a number of providers. The Pilot Program consortium application process encourages projects to centralize their implementation efforts and spread their administrative costs over all the health care providers in their network, which results in cost savings to the participants.[316] Pilot projects were required to apply as a network and to centralize their leadership by designating a project leader and project coordinators, which could be an eligible HCP or an entity responsible for handling the application process on behalf of eligible HCPs.[317] Centralizing the application and implementation process in this way has produced significant economies of scale and administrative cost savings for many of the Pilot projects.[318] Pilot project leaders took on the administrative tasks associated with applying for funding so that individual HCPs did not need to use their scarce administrative resources for this purpose.[319] The centralized structure also has reduced Pilot projects' need for consultants (as compared with the many Primary Program participants who often do

---

[309] *See* USAC Aug 2. Data Letter at 4.

[310] USAC May 30 Data Letter at 1-2. *See infra* Section V.A.

[311] *See* Aug. 4 Data Letter at 4.

[312] *See id.*; *see also* USAC May 30 Data Letter at 3.

[313] *See* Aug. 4 Data Letter at 4.

[314] *See id.*

[315] *See* USAC Observations Letter at 4.

[316] See USAC Observations Letter at 1-3.

[317] *See 2006 Pilot Program Order*, 21 FCC Rcd at 11111, 11116-17, paras. 3, 16-17.

[318] USAC Observations Letter at 1; PSPN Mar. 27 *Ex Parte* Letter at 2 (explaining that "individual members, especially in rural locations, often do not have the resources or time to navigate the RHC Primary Program process and it would be unimaginable that the RHC would want to receive literally hundreds of invoices per month from one local network, when the ability to bill as a consortium would be more efficient"); Cabarrus Health Alliance *et al.* Comments at 2.

[319] USAC Observations Letter at 1-2.

rely on consultants). In contrast, administrative costs have been higher for those projects that have chosen to decentralize the approach to contracting and invoicing.[320]

85. *Continuation of Institutional Knowledge.* Rural HCPs also commonly experience high staff turnover, so that the expertise in the application process is lost when staff departs.[321] Because a consortium approach encourages administrative resources and expertise to be centralized and shared, institutional knowledge is less likely to be lost through staff turnover.[322]

86. *Project Leadership and Contribution of Resources by Large Health Care Entities.* The consortium approach also enables rural HCPs to draw on the expertise and leadership of large health care entities, which often were the project leaders and the primary sources of technical and administrative expertise.[323] Project leaders typically are universities, state entities, hospitals, medical associations, or nonprofits with the mission of advancing telehealth and telemedicine initiatives.[324] These leaders often have the technical expertise and resources necessary to take advantage of Pilot project support and to facilitate the organization of groups of health care providers who could benefit from being part of a broadband network.[325] These leaders are also more likely to have access to the sophisticated information technology and other technical expertise necessary for network design, drafting of RFPs, integration of the networks with existing and planned telehealth applications, and training other sites.[326] This level of expertise is less often found in rural hospitals or clinics, so access to these resources within the larger health care network membership can be invaluable.[327] Additionally, large, usually urban, entities are more likely to have the necessary financial and administrative resources to pursue applications, given that the Pilot Program did not cover administrative expenses (see Section V.E below).[328]

87. *Improved Access to Health Care for Rural Patients Through Telemedicine and Health IT.* As discussed in detail above and below in Section V.B, rural health care providers that are part of a consortium benefit from being linked with larger HCPs, especially those in urban areas. Those linkages enable rural HCPs to access specialists through telemedicine and employ other telehealth applications, and thus to provide higher quality health care at lower cost. The involvement of physicians and other health care or health IT professionals in Pilot projects also helps projects to get off the ground quickly

---

[320] *Id.* at 2.

[321] NRHA Dec. 21 *Ex Parte* Letter at 1; NRHRC Dec. 27 *Ex Parte* Letter.

[322] *See* USAC Observations Letter at 1-3.

[323] Pilot Conference Call Mar. 13 *Ex Parte* Letter (PMHA *et al.*) at 2; USAC Observations Letter at 5.

[324] USAC Observations Letter at 1.

[325] Pilot Conference Call Mar. 13 *Ex Parte* Letter (PMHA *et al.)* at 3; USAC Observations Letter at 1; OHN Feb. 28 *Ex Parte* Letter at 7.

[326] USAC Observations Letter at 5.

[327] NRHA Dec. 21 *Ex Parte* Letter at 1 (discussing the difficulty that rural health care providers have in understanding their overall broadband needs, and further noting that IT budgets for rural hospitals and other rural health care providers are usually less than IT budgets for hospitals nationwide, which in turn are typically one-half to one-fourth of those in other industries); OHN Feb. 28 *Ex Parte* Letter at 7 (noting that many health care institutions in Oregon do not have a knowledgeable IT staff to support them in all phases of selection, installation, and use of broadband connections); John Gale Mar. 29 *Ex Parte* Letter at 2 (stating that informal networks to pool resources and technical expertise in order to support the implementation of electronic medical records were largely occurring among hospitals, not rural health clinics, but that rural health clinics could be affiliated with such hospitals).

[328] *See 2006 Pilot Program Order,* 21 FCC Rcd at 11115-16, paras. 14-15.

and to secure funding.[329] Health care professionals (particularly physicians) can play an important role in convincing others to invest in broadband and create broadband networks as a means to foster the use of telehealth applications – including telemedicine, electronic medical records, exchange of medical information, and training.[330] For example, Western New York Rural Health Education Center found that its Chief Information Officers and medical leadership were the champions of its network.[331] In some cases, the Pilot projects are being led by health care professionals who were using telemedicine or health information technology before becoming involved in the Pilot, and thus can show how broadband networks supported by the Pilot Program can be used to extend the benefits of their programs to smaller hospitals and clinics in rural areas.[332]

B.   Inclusion of Urban Providers

88.   The Pilot projects benefited significantly from the inclusion of urban HCPs in their networks. Unlike the Primary Program, the Commission permitted applicants to include public and not-for-profit urban locations in the Pilot projects, as long as the rural HCPs represented more than a *de minimis* number of the HCPs in the network.[333] As of January 31, 2012, all but 6 of the 50 active projects included at least one urban HCP.[334] The urban sites represented approximately 35 percent of the 2,107 Pilot project sites and approximately 35 percent of the funding commitments for all projects as of January 2012.[335] As noted above, the percentage of funds allocated to urban sites likely overstates the support flowing to urban sites in the Pilot Program because 100 percent of some shared expenses are attributed to urban locations, even though those expenses benefit the entire network.[336]

89.   Participation of urban sites in the Pilot Program provides many benefits for the Pilot projects. According to a number of Pilot projects, participation by urban sites has been instrumental to

---

[329] USAC Observations Letter at 2; Pilot Conference Call Mar. 26 *Ex Parte* Letter (AEN *et al.*) at 1; Colorado Feb. 28 *Ex Parte* Letter at 1.

[330] USAC Mar. 16 Site Visit Reports at 2, 6. *See also* Pilot Conference Call Mar. 16 *Ex Parte* Letter (ARCHIE *et al.*) at 1-2 (noting that physician involvement is key to broad telemedicine adoption); Telehealth Resource Center, Operation Tools: How Should Telemedicine be Introduced to Local Physicians?, *available at* http://www.telehealthresourcecenter.org/toolbox-module/introducing-telemedicine-services-community#how-can-the-local-providers-be-informed-of-the-ava (last visited June 15, 2012) (finding that a referring physician may be "skeptical of the value of telemedicine due to the concern about the potential loss of the doctor-patient relationship that is fostered in face-to-face care"); Lawrence Eron, *Telemedicine: The Future of Outpatient Therapy?*, Clinical Infectious Diseases, Vol: 51(S2), S224-S230, S229 (2010), *available at* http://cid.oxfordjournals.org/content/51/Supplement_2/S224.full.pdf+html (last visited June 15, 2012) (noting the concern of some physicians that telemedicine may foster "complacency regarding the risks and responsibilities—many of which are as yet unknown—that distant medical intervention, consultation, and diagnosis carry").

[331] *See* Pilot Conference Call Mar. 26 *Ex Parte* Letter (WNYRAHEC *et al.*) at 2.

[332] USAC Observations Letter at 2. *See also* Pilot Conference Call Mar. 26 *Ex Parte* Letter (AEN *et al.*) at 1 (noting that there was more interest in the Virginia Acute Stroke Telehealth project after initial sites showed that the proposed uses were viable); Pilot Conference Call Mar. 26 *Ex Parte* Letter (WNYRAHEC *et al.*) at 2 (describing that Geisinger Health System has already fully implemented EHRs and emphasizing the importance of getting the community together and involved to win their trust).

[333] *2006 Pilot Program Order*, 21 FCC Rcd at 11111, 11114, 11116, paras. 3, 10, 16; *see also 2007 Pilot Program Selection Order*, 22 FCC Rcd at 20368-69, 20384-85, paras. 19, 50.

[334] USAC Aug. 6 Data Letter at 2.

[335] USAC June 27 Data Letter at 1; USAC May 4 Data Letter at 3; USAC May 30 Data Letter at 2.

[336] USAC May 30 Data Letter at 2.

their individual success, and rural HCPs value their connections to urban hospitals.[337] These benefits include:

- Health Care Benefits:

    - *Access to Specialists.* Participation of urban sites enables rural providers to access medical specialists who might otherwise be unavailable or very distant.[338] Rural areas generally do not have the same access to specialist care (or even primary care) that urban areas have.[339] There is a shortage of specialists in rural areas, and rural health care providers can use broadband networks to connect to urban HCPs and obtain access to the medical specialists who work there. Telemedicine has allowed shortened waiting times at rural facilities for patients who need specialized medical care (often, hours rather than days).[340] Connections to urban locations also allow rural hospitals to move from a "patch and ship" mode – where they stabilize patients and then send them to urban hospitals – to keeping more patients in the rural hospital while consulting specialists remotely.[341] This not only can result in better patient care, it also can help rural hospitals financially.[342]

---

[337] *See, e.g.,* Pilot Conference Call Mar. 13 *Ex Parte* Letter (PMHA *et al.*) at 2 (group of five Pilot projects stated that urban HCP participation is "the key to the networks' success"); Colorado Feb. 28 *Ex Parte* Letter at 2 (stating that Colorado has created a 60 percent rural, 40 percent urban statewide health care network that "undergirds, complements, and strengthens the existing and necessary urban/rural interdependencies," and stating that supporting only rural sites fails to recognize the reality of urban/rural interdependencies); NOSORH Mar. 28 *Ex Parte* Letter at 1 (stating that in Minnesota, urban hospitals are typically the hubs of health care networks, and more and more rural hospitals are joining as spoke sites to those hubs); Pilot Conference Call Mar. 26 *Ex Parte* Letter (WNYRAHEC *et al.*) at 2-3 (WNYRAHEC stated that without its urban partners, it would be "building a road to nowhere").

[338] USAC Observations Letter at 5; PSPN Feb. 23 *Ex Parte* Letter at 1 (rural hospitals are "referring" sites, and the regional or tertiary hospitals are usually located in urban areas and serve as the "consulting" sites); OHN Feb. 28 *Ex Parte* Letter at 6-7 (stating that the subsidy for urban providers is critical to supporting integrated health care delivery, that rural/frontier providers are looking for improved access to urban specialists and resources to augment their dwindling clinical and operational resources, and that without the urban centers of excellence being on and actively using the network connection, there would be no value to the rural/frontier providers in connecting; also noting that in Oregon, one university hospital and two pediatric hospitals in Portland provide much of the specialty care to rural facilities); Pilot Conference Call Mar. 13 *Ex Parte* Letter (PMHA *et al.*) at 2-3 (group of five Pilot projects stated that rural HCPs value their connection to urban hospitals and their instant access to specialized care); Pilot Conference Call Mar. 26 *Ex Parte* Letter (AEN *et al.*) at 1 (group of five Pilot projects stated that the inclusion of urban sites in the Pilot Program was critical to providing specialty care, because of the shortage of specialists in urban areas); USAC Mar. 16 Site Visit Reports at 14 (Henry County Health Center in Iowa reports that it primarily uses its broadband connection for radiology services, as there is no radiologist on staff); USAC Apr. 27 Site Visit Reports at 3 (patients at the Coffee Walk-in Clinic in southeastern Georgia can see specialists in Atlanta, Savannah, or Jacksonville that they would otherwise have no access to or would have to travel several hours in each direction to see).

[339] *See* NRHRC Dec. 27 *Ex Parte* Letter at 2; OHN Feb. 28 *Ex Parte* Letter at 7; USAC Observations Letter at 5; Pilot Conference Call Mar. 16 *Ex Parte* Letter at 1-2 (ARCHIE *et al.*) at 1 (inclusion of urban sites in the Pilot Program was critical to providing specialty care, because of the shortage of specialists in rural areas).

[340] *See, e.g.,* USAC Mar. 16 Site Visit Reports at 11.

[341] Pilot Project Conference Call Mar. 16 *Ex Parte* Letter (ARCHIE *et al.*) at 1-2. *See also* Pilot Project Conference Call Mar. 25 *Ex Parte* Letter (WNYRAHEC *et al.*) at 2; USAC Observations Letter at 5; Pilot Conference Call Mar. 13 *Ex Parte* Letter (PHMA *et al.*) at 2; OHN Feb. 28 *Ex Parte* Letter at 7 (no value for rural providers to connect to their network without the urban centers on the network since rural HCPs "are looking for improved access to urban specialists and resources to augment their dwindling clinical and operational resources").

[342] Pilot Conference Call Mar. 13 *Ex Parte* Letter (PHMA *et al.*) at 2-3, ORHP Apr. 10 *Ex Parte* Letter at 2.

Some experts believe that primary care physicians will be more likely to stay in rural areas if they can draw on those urban resources via broadband connections.[343]

- *Health Care Cost Savings*. As discussed above, and as demonstrated through the implemented Pilot projects, there is an enormous potential for health care cost savings if rural health care providers can use telemedicine to keep patients in their rural communities, through reduced hospital stays and lower transportation costs. This may also in some instances produce additional revenue streams for the health care providers. Leveraging the resources in urban areas to benefit rural providers is an efficient means to keep patients in rural communities.[344]

- *Training of Health Care Personnel in Rural Areas*. Broadband connections to urban hospitals and universities can provide opportunities for training and for transfer of expertise to rural areas.[345] There is a shortage of trained health professional and health IT experts in rural areas.[346] Broadband connections to urban locations can deliver necessary expertise and training to those rural areas, thus accelerating their adoption of medical best practices, as well as implementation of electronic health records and other health IT applications.[347]

- Administrative Benefits:

  - *Leadership of Consortia*. As noted above, the organizers and leaders of many of the projects are urban entities – especially hospitals and university medical centers.[348] For example, the lead entity for HUBNet is Avera Health in Sioux Falls, South Dakota, the lead entity for the PSPN is the Medical University of South Carolina in Charleston, and the lead entity for the Iowa Rural Health Telecommunications Program is the Mercy Health System in Des Moines.[349] In some cases, the urban entities already owned or led

---

[343] *See supra* para. 70.

[344] *See supra* Section IV.C.

[345] *See supra* n. 251 and accompanying text.

[346] *See supra* para. 63.

[347] Pilot Conference Call Mar. 26 *Ex Parte* Letter (WNYRAHEC *et al.*) at 2-3 (WNYRAHEC stated that it is important that urban medical centers participate because creativity and innovation is located there); NRHRC Dec. 27 *Ex Parte* Letter at 1 (explaining that due to the current health IT workforce shortage, vendors are short staffed and conducting much of the training for implementation of EHR systems over videoconference links, which HCPs need at least a 5 Mbps connection to access); USAC Mar. 16 Site Visit Reports at 6 (explaining that Avera provides participating rural HCPs with 24/7 order review for patients in outlying hospitals, which is necessary because most rural HCPs do not have pharmacists on staff, and that the E-Pharmacy program has allowed Avera Flandreau, a rural hospital, to meet stage one of meaningful use requirements).

[348] USAC Observations Letter at 4-5 (stating that for most Pilot projects, urban centers provided necessary leadership to bring disparate stakeholders together, given that stakeholders include different health care disciplines and market competitors).

[349] USAC Mar. 16 Site Visit Reports at 5, 9, 13. Examples of other such projects include the California Telehealth Network (spearheaded by the University of California system and managed initially through the University of California Davis Health System); Rocky Mountain HealthNet (coordinated by the Colorado Behavioral Healthcare Council, which is based in Denver); and Colorado Health Care Connections (sponsored and housed at the Colorado Hospital Association in the Denver metropolitan areas). *See* Quarterly Report of the California Telehealth Network, WC Docket No. 02-60, at 4 (filed Apr. 27, 2012); Quarterly Report of the Rocky Mountain Healthcare Network,

(continued . . .)

networks of rural hospitals and clinics when they made the decision to apply as a Pilot project. The Pilot projects often added additional sites to these pre-existing networks, or created state-wide or multi-state "networks of networks."[350]

- *Sources of Technical Expertise.* The technical expertise necessary to design networks, develop RFPs, and manage the IT aspects of the network is often located at urban sites. Urban sites also often have greater expertise in telemedicine, electronic health records, Health IT, computer systems, and other broadband telehealth applications.[351]

- *Financial Resources.* Many of the Pilot projects have depended on the financial and human resources of urban entities to absorb the administrative costs of participation in the Pilot, such as the cost of planning and organizing the Pilot applications, applying for funding, preparing RFPs, contracting for services, and implementing the Pilot projects. Those expenses are not eligible for support under the Pilot Program.[352]

- Technical Benefits:

  - *Efficiency of Network Design.* In addition, network design in many cases has been more efficient and less costly in the Pilot Program than in the Primary Program, because the Pilot Program funds urban locations. Under the Primary Program, circuits are only eligible for funding if one end of the circuit terminates at an eligible rural entity, which

(. . . continued from previous page) ———————————————
WC Docket No. 02-60, at 1 (filed Apr. 26, 2012); Quarterly Report of Colorado Health Care Connections, WC Docket No. 02-60, at 2 (filed Apr. 26, 2012).

[350] *See, e.g.,* HUBNet Program Application, WC Docket No. 02-60 (filed May 7, 2007) at 5-7; PSPN Program Application, WC Docket No. 02-60 (filed May 4, 2007) at 9-17; IRHTP Program Application, WC Docket No. 02-60 (filed May 7, 2007) at 10-11. *See also* Pilot Conference Call Mar. 16 *Ex Parte* Letter at 1-2 (ARCHIE *et al.*) at 2 (several projects described their ultimate goal as achieving a "network of networks" linking pre-existing networks of health care providers together, sometimes with planned state-wide coverage); NOSORH Mar. 28 *Ex Parte* Letter at 1 (in Minnesota, the Pilot Program instigated the creation of a "network of networks" in which five different networks joined together to form one umbrella network).

[351] *See* NRHA Dec. 21 *Ex Parte* Letter at 1 (describing difficulty rural health care providers have in understanding their overall broadband needs, and the relative paucity of rural health providers' IT budgets); OHN Feb. 28, 2012 *Ex Parte* Letter at 7 (noting that in Oregon, many health care institutions do not have a knowledgeable IT staff); John Gale Mar. 29 *Ex Parte* Letter at 1-2 (stating that the typical rural health clinic has an average of 2.7 physicians and 1-1.5 mid-level practitioners, and that the majority of RHC practitioners must see five to six patients per hour to remain financially sustainable, leaving little time to devote to technological upgrades or meetings with consultants); USAC Observations Letter at 5 (urban centers typically have IT expertise and technology typically not found in rural areas, and the participation of urban HCPs in the Pilot Program, especially the urban leadership, has resulted in urban entities providing their IT expertise to their rural counterparts to assist with connectivity issues, training rural staff how to utilize the new resources, and equipment installation); Pilot Conference Call Mar. 13 *Ex Parte* Letter (PMHA *et al.*) at 2-3 (group of five Pilot projects stated that urban HCPs have provided technical support to rural HCPs and trained some of their IT staff, which has led to an improved rural HCP workforce).

[352] Pilot Conference Call Mar. 13 *Ex Parte* Letter (PMHA *et al.*) at 2-3 (group of five Pilot projects stated that many rural HCPs rely on urban sites in their network to pay for their networks' administrative expenses); Colorado Feb. 28 *Ex Parte* Letter at 1 (citing "the recognition by urban hospitals of the common good provided by this project and their willingness to provide financial support" as a success factor); Pilot Conference Call Mar. 26 *Ex Parte* Letter (WNYRAHEC *et al.*) at 2-3 (Bacon County noted it was able to purchase its (non-RHC-eligible) telehealth equipment through a grant from an urban hospital in its network); USAC Mar. 16 Site Visit Reports at 6 (rural ER nurses can connect to urban site with the push of a button, and the urban "presence" allows rural nurses to focus on providing patient care without worrying about the paperwork, which the urban site handles).

can incentivize HCPs to maximize funding by ensuring that all connections within the network terminate at an eligible rural entity.[353] As a technical and financial matter, this can lead to less efficient network design. For example, it may be more efficient to design the middle-mile component of a regional or statewide network by using connections between urban sites. Pilot projects were able to design their networks with maximum network efficiency in mind, since there is no negative impact on funding from including urban nodes within the network.[354]

90. Some Pilot projects observe that urban locations might not have been willing to assume leadership roles, taken on the administrative burdens, or contributed technical expertise if they had not also been allowed to obtain discounts on their broadband connections to rural sites.[355] USAC notes that many urban locations were able to serve as hubs for Pilot Program networks because they were eligible to receive funding to purchase equipment that allowed them to establish the network connections and any financial hardship associated with purchasing equipment was no longer a barrier to entry.[356] Participants indicate that urban hospitals are often as hard pressed for available funding as rural hospitals.[357]

C.   Ownership of Broadband Facilities Versus Purchased Services

91. The Pilot Program was designed to fund broadband infrastructure deployment and the creation of broadband networks of health care providers.[358] The Pilot projects have achieved these goals, though not usually by owning the broadband facilities. In the *2007 Pilot Program Selection Order*, the Commission permitted Pilot projects to create their networks by leasing services or constructing and owning their own broadband networks.[359] For the most part, HCPs chose to assemble their networks through purchasing services, including through indefeasible rights of use (IRU) or other long-term arrangements, rather than by owning and operating the networks themselves, as discussed above in Section III.F.[360] In effect, they have demonstrated that dedicated health care networks do not require

---

[353] USAC Observations Letter at 5.

[354] *Id.*

[355] Pilot Conference Call Mar. 13 *Ex Parte* Letter (PMHA *et al.*) at 3 (summarizing call with five Pilot project representatives, who stated in relevant part that due to the current economic environment, budgets are tight for urban HCPs, and it may be difficult for urban HCPs to continue to provide support to rural HCPs in their networks if they are ineligible to receive RHC program funding themselves); PSPN Feb. 23 *Ex Parte* Letter at 1 (stating that urban hospitals, which serve as "consulting" sites for rural hospitals in telemedicine, are often as hard-pressed for available funding as the rural hospitals and cannot bear the non-discounted costs of participation in the networks, and without their participation, vital links in the chain of health care are missing).

[356] USAC Observations Letter at 5.

[357] Pilot Conference Call Mar. 13 *Ex Parte* Letter (PMHA *et al.*) at 3 (summarizing call with five Pilot project representatives, who stated in relevant part that due to the current economic environment, budgets are tight for urban HCPs, and it may be difficult for urban HCPs to continue to provide support to rural HCPs in their networks if they are ineligible to receive RHC program funding themselves); PSPN Feb. 23 *Ex Parte* Letter at 1 (stating that urban hospitals, which serve as "consulting" sites for rural hospitals in telemedicine, are often as hard-pressed for available funding as the rural hospitals and cannot bear the non-discounted costs of participation in the networks, and without their participation, vital links in the chain of health care are missing).

[358] *2006 Pilot Program Order*, 21 FCC Rcd at 11111, 11114, paras. 1, 10.

[359] *2007 Pilot Program Selection Order*, 22 FCC Rcd at 20397-98, para. 74.

HCP *ownership* of those networks, although funding of network construction and upgrades can be essential in order to provide rural HCPs to have access to broadband where it is not already available.[361]

92. There may be several reasons why Pilot projects have not generally chosen to construct and own their own broadband facilities. First, running a network is a complex and technical task, and using third-party services can be simpler.[362] Second, it has not always proven necessary for projects to own the facilities in order to obtain broadband deployment to sites previously unserved by high-speed connections. In many cases, service providers have laid fiber and made other investments where necessary to enable them to provide the services requested.[363] Third, through long-term contracts, prepaid leases, and IRUs, projects have been able to obtain low prices for long terms as well as high service quality and reliability and virtual private network configurations.[364] Thus, for many projects it has been unnecessary for the Pilot projects to own the network facilities in order to secure good pricing and high service quality. Fourth, by purchasing services as opposed to owning the network, projects can obtain the underlying services from a range of service providers, and thus can obtain a broader geographic reach, coordinated services, and often lower prices.[365] Fifth, purchasing services allows HCPs to avoid the risk and cost of owning facilities.[366] Finally, HCPs are not permitted to sell, resell, or

[360] *See supra* Section III.F; USAC Observations Letter at 7-8. Whether using owned or leased facilities, the projects are still subject to requirements that they use the networks for health care purposes, that they not resell services over the networks, and that they obtain a "fair share" contribution from ineligible sites on their networks. *2007 Pilot Program Selection Order*, 22 FCC Rcd at 20416, para. 107.

[361] *See generally* Section III.F above; USAC Observations Letter at 7-8.

[362] *See, e.g.,* Colorado Feb. 28 *Ex Parte* Letter at 2 (Colorado projects did not want to divert resources away from their core competency, health care, into communications operations); Pilot Conference Call Mar. 13 *Ex Parte* Letter (PMHA *et al.*) at 3 (group of Pilot projects stating that their core competencies did not include constructing and owning networks, and that they preferred to purchase services); Pilot Conference Call Mar. 26 *Ex Parte* Letter (AEN *et al.*) at 2 (noting comment that most stakeholders prefer not to own the physical facilities comprising their network, but would rather defer to service providers that have experience and expertise in these matters to complete any build out, and stating that in cases where construction is necessary, the HCP may issue one RFP for construction and a second RFP for an experienced entity to manage the network on behalf of the health care provider); Pilot Conference Call Mar. 16 *Ex Parte* Letter (ARCHIE *et al.*) at 3 (stating that while the Pilot Program helped prompt the deployment of fiber or other high capacity facilities to many HCP sites where such facilities were not previously available, health care providers do not want to own the network facilities).

[363] *See supra* Section III.F; USAC Observations Letter at 7-8; USAC May 30 Data Letter at 3-4. *See also, e.g.,* OHN Feb. 28 *Ex Parte* Letter at 3 (stating that OHN's leased services model stimulated the deployment of 86.41 miles of new middle-mile connectivity across the farthest reaches of Oregon, and utilized 151.06 miles of existing infrastructure).

[364] *See supra* Sections III.E-III.H; USAC Observations Letter at 7-8; USAC May 30 Data Letter at 3-4; USAC Aug. 2 Data Letter at 4-5.

[365] USAC May 30 Data Letter at 1- 3; USAC May 4 Data Letter at App. C; Colorado Feb. 28 *Ex Parte* Letter at 2 (by using leased services and leveraging existing communications infrastructure, Colorado projects were able to include far more providers than if they had built and owned their own network); OHN Feb. 28 *Ex Parte* Letter at 1 (stating that OHN's multi-vendor leased line network framework helped utilize the existing state fiber infrastructure while creating the highest level of competition possible, allowing smaller local carriers to compete directly and fairly with larger providers, which subsequently resulted in OHN's members receiving the most competitive bids (reduced costs) possible); Pilot Conference Call Mar. 13 *Ex Parte* Letter (PMHA *et al.*) at 3 (group of Pilot projects stating that leasing services allowed the projects to reach many more health care providers than the construction options).

[366] *See, e.g.,* Colorado Feb. 28 *Ex Parte* Letter at 2 (stating that CTN's core competency is health care, and they did not want to divert resources into telecommunications operations); OHN Feb. 28 *Ex Parte* Letter at 1 (stating that

(continued . . .)

otherwise transfer communications services or network capacity purchased through the rural health care mechanism.[367] Although ineligible HCPs can still participate in networks if they pay a "fair share" of network costs, some Pilot projects have had difficulty in determining the appropriate fair share that ineligible for-profit network members should pay.[368]

93. Nevertheless, the ability to use program funds for some construction, even in limited circumstances, benefited projects. Although the Pilot projects generally chose not to own their broadband facilities, some did use Pilot project funding to enable service providers to build broadband facilities, or to upgrade existing facilities, as discussed in Section III.F above.[369] In many cases, last-mile and even middle mile broadband facilities do not exist in some of the rural areas that Pilot projects serve, so construction was an important element in providing broadband capability to HCPs located in those areas.[370] Long-term contracts, prepaid leases, IRUs, and similar arrangements can help provide incentives for communications service providers to build or upgrade network facilities where needed.[371] Experience thus far suggests that these arrangements also provided HCPs with lower rates, higher bandwidth, greater service quality, and long-term stability of pricing.[372] In addition, some Pilot projects have taken advantage of the Pilot Program's broader definition of "eligible expenses" (compared with the Primary Program), which includes construction costs. Two Pilot projects own their entire network, and a number of other projects have decided to own parts of the network, or to own the Network Operations Center (NOC).[373] Those projects concluded that ownership of the facilities would bring significant price and other benefits.[374] In addition, others observe that the existence of a last-resort option enabling the HCPs to construct and own their own broadband network facilities may help encourage bidders to respond to RFPs with more favorable offerings and lower prices, and that such an option gives HCPs the ability to construct broadband connections in situations in which no provider is willing to do so.[375]

(. . . continued from previous page) ─────────────────────────────
utilizing existing fiber infrastructure to create a leased line network granted OHN a lot less administrative burden and overhead versus owning the actual equipment and fiber connection).

[367] Section 254(h)(3) of the 1996 Act provides that "telecommunications services and network capacity provided to a public institutional telecommunications under this subsection may not be sold, resold, or otherwise transferred by such user in consideration for money or any other thing of value." 47 C.F.R. § 254(h)(3). *See also* 47 C.F.R. § 54.617; *Universal Service First Report and Order*, 12 FCC Rcd at 8795, para. 33.

[368] *See* Pilot Conference Call Mar. 26 *Ex Parte* Letter (AEN et al.) at 3; *2006 Pilot Program Order*, 21 FCC Rcd at 11116, para. 17. For example, Pilot projects that wanted to include ineligible sites on a Pilot-owned network would need to determine, with USAC, how to handle such issues as fair share, incremental costs, excess capacity and excess bandwidth. *See* Pilot Program Frequently Asked Questions, *available at* http://www.fcc.gov/encyclopedia/rural-health-care-pilot-program.

[369] *See also* USAC Observations Letter at 7-8.

[370] Pilot Conference Call Mar. 16 *Ex Parte* Letter (ARCHIE *et al.*) at 3 (stating that ownership of newly constructed facilities only makes economic sense where there are gaps in availability).

[371] *See* USAC Observations Letter at 4.

[372] *Id.*; *see also* USAC Aug. 2 Data Letter at 4.

[373] USAC Observations Letter at 7-8.

[374] *See, e.g.,* Pilot Conference Call Mar. 26 *Ex Parte* Letter (WNYRAHEC *et al.*) at 1 (noting that having a private fiber network as part of the larger network helped St. Joseph's to control costs and ensure long-term success, as it could be cost-prohibitive to buy from a carrier the 1 to 10 Gbps connections needed to move medical images).

[375] *See, e.g.,* HIEM *Ex Parte* Letter at 2 (stating that HIEM's network would be a small fraction of what it is now if HIEM had simply leased facilities from the outset, and arguing that the Commission should retain the option for

(continued . . .)

D.   Funding of Network Design Studies

94. As mentioned previously, the scope of eligible expenses is broader in the Pilot Program than the Primary Program and included network design studies.[376] However, those projects that decided to take advantage of the opportunity to have network design studies conducted before they started to build their networks may have been delayed by doing so.[377] The six projects that have invoiced USAC for completing network design studies have gone through the Pilot Program administrative process to request funding twice, once for the network design studies and a second time to solicit bids to build the network.[378] Five of these six projects have experienced significant delays in implementing their networks, as illustrated in the figure below.[379]

Figure 18 – Pilot Projects that Conducted Network Design Studies[380]

Pilot Project Name	Amount Committed for Network Design Study	Percent of Original Award Committed (As of Jan. 31, 2012)
Oregon Health Network	$174,650	83.63%
New England Telehealth Consortium	$746,134	3.02%
Louisiana Department of Hospitals	$399,904	2.51%
Erlanger Health System	$38,250	1.74%
Arkansas Telehealth Network	$338,827	8.03%
Alaska eHealth Network	$208,888	2.00%

E.   Administrative Expenses

95. Some Pilot projects expressed frustration that administrative expenses are not an eligible expense in the Pilot Program, and several have suggested such expenses should be supported.[381] Such

(. . . continued from previous page) ————————————
program participants to construct network facilities, as removing that option from competitive bidding will change how incumbent carriers approach the bid process).

[376] See 2006 Pilot Program Order, 21 FCC Rcd at 11111, para. 1, 11115-16, paras. 14-15; see also 2007 Pilot Program Selection Order, 22 FCC Rcd at 20397-98, para. 74.

[377] See USAC Aug. 2 Data Letter at 3.

[378] Id.

[379] USAC Observations Letter at 8. The sixth project sought funding for its Network Operations Center (NOC) design only. Because the project only designed its NOC, it was able to lease lines to implement its network simultaneously with the design of the NOC. It then issued an RFP for the NOC after the lines were in place and the NOC design was completed, resulting in no delay. Id.

[380] USAC Aug. 9 Data Letter at App. C.

[381] Colorado Feb. 28 Ex Parte Letter at 2, Pilot Conference Call Mar. 26 Ex Parte Letter (AEN et al.) at 2 (discussing the difficulties faced by Pilot projects in raising sufficient administrative funds to engage stakeholders and pursue the complex application and proposal process, and noting that one Pilot project had invested $500,000 in administrative expenses due to the number of stakeholders involved, while another project had a seven figure budget for administrative expenses). Some Pilot Projects also noted that the exclusion of administrative expenses as an eligilble expenses was hardship on the projects. See Pilot Conference Call Mar. 13 Ex Parte Letter (PMHA et al.) at 2 (stating that seeking funds to cover administrative expenses caused projects significant delay in getting their networks started, and that it was difficult for projects to come up with their own funds to pay for their own administrative expenses until their networks were built); Pilot Conference Call Mar. 16 Ex Parte Letter (ARCHIE et al.) at 1 (without funding for administrative expenses, it is hard to find funding to pull together a network of eligible HCPs, develop the proposals, and pursue the application process, especially given the cash-strapped position of many rural HCPs).

non-reimbursable costs include project design, identifying potential HCP participants, preparing application materials, obtaining letters of agency, preparing RFPs, and working with USAC to put together necessary application materials and associated documentation. For some Pilot projects, it came as a surprise that administrative costs were not covered, especially for those who were familiar with grant programs, which generally do cover such overhead costs. Many projects have observed that the administrative, technical, and communication requirements to participate in the program are substantial and require a staff that has marketing, communications, legal, healthcare, finance, policy, and/or IT knowledge and expertise.[382] As a result, some projects have spent large amounts on administrative expenses. For example, Oregon Health Network estimated that it spends $930,000 annually on administrative expenses, and another Pilot project states that it has invested up to $500,000 in administrative expenses as of February 2012.[383] Western New York Rural Area Health Education Center also notes that its direct administrative expenses are $65,000.[384] Indiana Telehealth Network (ITN) initially received a $250,000 grant from the Indiana Office of Community and Rural Affairs for ineligible administrative costs.[385] However, as of 2011, the ITN now covers administrative costs by charging participating hospitals and other rural health care facilities $2,400 and $1,200 respectively per year.[386] Other projects also fund administrative expenses through membership fees.[387] As noted above in Section V.B, many relied on the urban providers in their networks to help support their administrative expenses, by donating resources, both personnel and otherwise.

F.   Requirement for Sustainability Plans

96. *Sustainability Plan Requirement.* Many Pilot projects expressed difficulty in predicting their long-term sustainability, and some plan on relying on sources outside of their networks for long-term funding.[388] Before they can receive Pilot Program support, projects were required to submit sustainability plans detailing their plans to ensure the long-term success of rural health care networks after the Pilot program ceases to exist and their plans to prevent wasteful allocation of limited universal service funds.[389] Sustainability plans were required in the *2007 Pilot Program Selection Order*, and in

---

[382] OHN Feb. 28 *Ex* Parte Letter at 6; *see also* Pilot Conference Call Mar. 13 *Ex Parte* Letter (PMHA *et al.*) at 2; Pilot Conference Call Mar. 16 *Ex Parte* Letter (ARCHIE *et al.*) at 2 (explaining that it was difficult to find funds to pay for administrative expenses, which caused delay"); Colorado Feb. 28 *Ex Parte* Letter at 2 (stating that even with the efficiencies of the consortium approach, the two Colorado Pilot projects experienced a substantial administrative burden to respond to program requirements, and noting that since the Pilot Program enabled creation of a statewide health care network, there was no pre-existing entity that had responsibility and a concomitant budget).

[383] Pilot Conference Call Mar. 26 *Ex Parte* Letter (WNYRAHEC *et al.*) at 3 (providing information on administrative expenses incurred by Pilot projects, which ranged from $42,000 to $930,000 annually, depending on the project); Pilot Conference Call Mar. 26 *Ex Parte* Letter (AEN *et al.*) at 2.

[384] Pilot Conference Call Mar. 26 *Ex Parte* Letter (WNYRAHEC *et al.*) at 3.

[385] Quarterly Report of Indiana Telehealth Network, WC Docket No. 02-60 (filed Jan. 27, 2012) at 34.

[386] *Id.*

[387] Pilot Conference Call Mar. 26 *Ex Parte* Letter (WNYRAHEC *et al.*) at 3; Quarterly Report of Pacific Broadband Telehealth Demonstration Project, WC Docket No. 02-60 (filed Jan. 29, 2012) at 16.

[388] *See, e.g.,* Pilot Conference Call Mar. 26 *Ex Parte* Letter (AEN *et al.*) at 2. Some rural HCPs stated that it can be difficult to secure funding for broadband connections, even with a universal service discount. *See* Pilot Conference Call Mar. 16 *Ex Parte* Letter (ARCHIE *et al.*) at 1; NRHRC Dec. 27 *Ex Parte* Letter at 2 (many critical access hospitals and small rural hospitals are experiencing negative margins and facing increased difficulties in accessing capital); John Gale Mar. 29 *Ex Parte* Letter at 2.

[389] *2007 Pilot Program Selection Order,* 22 FCC Rcd at 20388, paras. 54, 108.

April 2009 the Commission provided more details about what projects should include in their sustainability plans.[390] Among other things, the Commission explained that sustainability plans should include a description of how a project will be self-sustaining in the future, network ownership and membership arrangements, and future sources of support such as a project's reliance on their participating providers, government funding and/or private donors to ensure continued financial viability for a specific period of time.[391] The Commission also recommended that a demonstration of sustainability for ten years would be generally appropriate, but that the plan should be commensurate with the investments made with Pilot Program funds.[392]

97. Pilot projects anticipate relying upon a variety of internal and external funding sources to achieve sustainability, including government and private organization grants, as demonstrated by the figure below. Nearly 10 percent of Pilot projects declared in their sustainability plans their intent to rely exclusively on participating health care providers,[393] and over half of the Pilot projects plan to look to both participating providers and anticipated cost savings/new revenue streams to achieve network sustainability.[394] Some Pilot projects include in their sustainability plans the projected cost savings they expect to derive from achieving economies of scale.[395] Several Pilot projects also stated that enhanced telehealth capabilities will reduce travel, training, and operational costs – cost savings that can help project sites offset network connectivity costs.[396] Pilot projects also highlighted the potential revenue stream telehealth applications may provide participating entities, particularly with respect to tele-psychiatry services.[397] Figure 19, below, lists the categories of sustainability plan sources and the frequency with which Pilot projects intend to rely on these categories in their sustainability plans.

---

[390] Rural Health Care Pilot Program: Frequently Asked Questions and Answers, *available at* http://www.fcc.gov/encyclopedia/rural-health-care-pilot-program (last viewed June 15, 2012). These elements included how projects would obtain a 15% funding match for their project; the project's projected sustainability period; principal factors the project considered in demonstrating their sustainability, their terms of membership in the network (*i.e.,* agreements made by network members to enter into network, financial commitments made by proposed members of the network, membership fees, financing of excess bandwidth), sources of future support, management of excess capacity (if applicable), and the ownership structure of the network. *Id.*

[391] *Id.*

[392] *Id.*

[393] Quarterly Report of Greater Minnesota Telehealth Broadband Initiative, WC Docket No. 02-60, at 14 (filed Jan. 31, 2012); Quarterly Report of Illinois Rural HealthNet Consortium, WC Docket No. 02-60, at 19-20 (filed Jan. 24, 2012); Quarterly Report of Michigan Public Health Institute, WC Docket No. 02-60, at 30-33 (filed Jan. 30, 2012); Quarterly Report of Rural Wisconsin Healthcare Cooperative Information Technology Network, WC Docket No. 02-60, at 43-44 (filed Jan. 31, 2012).

[394] This information is based on staff review of Pilot participants' 2011-2012 quarterly reports.

[395] *See supra* Section IV.C.2.

[396] *See id.*

[397] *See id.*

Figure 19 – Sustainability Plan Sources[398]

Sustainability Plan Sources (Other than FCC Support)	Count	Percentage
Participants; New revenue and/or Cost savings	26	52%
Participants; Govt. funding	5	10%
Participants	4	8%
No details provided	4	8%
Participants; New revenue and/or Cost savings; Govt. funding	3	6%
Participants; New revenue and/or Cost savings; Govt. funding; Private donors	2	4%
New revenue streams and/or Cost savings	2	4%
New revenue streams and/or Cost savings; Govt. funding	2	4%
Participants; Govt. funding; Private donors	2	4%
Total	50	100%

98. While Figure 19 reflects significant planning on the part of the Pilot projects, several projects noted that accurately predicting a long term sustainability plan was a "best guess at most."[399] Further, as many networks are not yet operational, on-going costs of the network may be difficult to predict accurately. Some Pilot projects voice concerns about submitting plans that attempt to forecast their sustainability for more than five years, given the rapid and unpredictable changes in healthcare needs and broadband technology.[400] Additionally, one project notes that it was difficult to develop a sustainability plan because that requirement was not part of the original application.[401] Nevertheless, USAC notes that "the benefits of the sustainability plan show thoughtful planning as to the HCPs planned network use, demonstration of administrative function necessary to maintain the network, and a demonstration of a financial model that would ensure sustainability."[402]

99. *Continued Reliance on FCC Support by Pilot Participants.* Over half of the Pilot project sustainability plans reported their intent to rely on FCC support in the future. However, a sizeable minority (38 percent) of all projects did not mention the potential for continued Primary Program support.[403] While this omission may be due to a lack of awareness, it may also be attributable to participants' uncertainty with respect to the form that continued FCC support will take. For example, the Adirondack-Champlain Telemedicine Information Network stated that "[a]t this time we have not included any budget references for sites that meet the eligibility requirements for the regular RHC funding program . . . [and] will apply for funding at a future date once we determine how the Primary Program will be restructured."[404] Likewise, Heartland Unified Broadband Network laid out three sustainability plan scenarios in the event that either the Primary Program provided an 85 percent

---

[398] This information is based on staff review of Pilot participants' 2011-2012 quarterly reports.

[399] *See, e.g.,* Quarterly Report of Southwest Telehealth Access Grid (SWTAG), WC Docket No. 02-60, at 17 (filed Jan. 27, 2012).

[400] Pilot Conference Call Mar. 26 *Ex Parte* Letter (AEN *et al.*) at 2.

[401] *Id.* at 2.

[402] USAC Observations Letter at 5.

[403] This information is based on staff review of Pilot participants' 2011-2012 quarterly reports.

[404] Quarterly Report of Adirondack Champlain Telemedicine Information Network (ACTION), WC Docket No. 02-60, at 17 (filed Jan. 20, 2012).

discount rate, maintained current funding levels, or if all funding for rural healthcare providers was phased out.[405]

G.   Multi-Year Commitments (Waiver of Annual Filing Requirement)

100.   Some Pilot projects identified the waiver of the annual filing requirement as beneficial. In the Primary Program, applicants must reapply to the program annually because they can only receive a funding commitment for the 12 months of the funding year.[406]   In contrast, the *2007 Pilot Program Selection Order* waived the annual filing requirement for Pilot projects,[407] which enables USAC to issue funding commitments based on the length of the contract (initial contract term only). The waiver of the annual filing requirement has created administrative efficiencies for USAC and the Pilot projects, including a reduction of hundreds of forms Pilot projects would otherwise have had to complete each year. It also has given projects incentives to sign long-term contracts that allowed them to lock in stable prices, and reduced the number of funding requests USAC had to review.[408]   North Carolina Telehealth Network notes that it is helpful that sites in the Pilot Program are guaranteed funding over the long-term, as compared to the Primary Program, where participants must seek funding approval every year (except in the case of "evergreen contracts").[409]

H.   Flat-Rate Discount

101.   Many of the Pilot Program participants appreciate the administrative simplicity and funding certainty provided by the Pilot Program's single, flat-rate discount for eligible infrastructure, purchase of services and other expenses.[410]   In the Primary Program, rural health care provider funding for telecommunications services is based on either the urban/rural price differential or on "mileage based support."[411]   In contrast, in the Pilot Program, funding is determined on a flat percentage discount for eligible services.[412]

102.   Projects identify three ways in which the flat-rate discount approach is helpful. First, they say it has reduced the complexity of participating in the Pilot Program, particularly from the

---

[405] Quarterly Report of Heartland Unified Broadband Network (HUBNet), WC Docket No. 02-60, at 57 (filed Jan. 30, 2012).

[406] 47 C.F.R. § 54.623(d).

[407] *2007 Pilot Program Selection Order,* 22 FCC Rcd at 20405-6, para. 86.

[408] USAC Observations Letter at 4.

[409] Pilot Conference Call Mar. 13 *Ex Parte* Letter (PMHA *et al.*) at 3.

[410] *See* Pilot Conference Call Mar. 13 *Ex Parte* Letter (PMHA *et al.*) at 3; *see also* Pilot Conference Call Mar. 26 *Ex Parte* Letter (AEN *et al.*) at 3; Pilot Conference Call Mar. 26 *Ex Parte* Letter (WNYRAHEC *et al.*) at 4.

[411] 47 C.F.R. §§ 54.605, 54.607, 54.609; USAC Observations Letter at 6. The Primary Program provides support for telecommunications services based on the difference between the rural and urban rate for non-mileage based charges or for the applicable distance-based charges (minus the Standard Urban Distance (SUD)) for the distance between the rural health care provider and the farthest point on the jurisdictional boundary of the largest city in the health care provider's state. If an eligible rural HCP chooses to connect to a point beyond this Maximum Allowable Distance (MAD), it must pay the appropriate unsupported rate for any distance-based charges incurred beyond the MAD. *See* USAC Rural Health Care FAQs, *available at* http://www.usac.org/rhc/about/getting-started/faqs.aspx (last visited June 8, 2012). The SUD is a mileage allowance for urban areas. There is a single SUD for each state. See USAC Rural Health Care Standard Urban Distance, *available at* https://www.rhc.universalservice.org/applicants/sud.asp (last visited June 8, 2012).

[412] *See 2007 Pilot Program Selection Order*, 22 FCC Rcd at 20361, para. 2.

perspective of consortium applicants, and has given them more certainty with respect to the discount level they can expect. Pilot Program participants are not required to calculate funding based on the urban/rural price differential and thus do not have to obtain pricing information to determine the urban/rural differential.[413] Calculating support for high-bandwidth circuits, like those supported by the Pilot Program, is particularly complex in the Primary Program because it often requires a complicated calculation of the Maximum Allowable Distance or Standard Urban Distance to determine mileage based support.[414] In addition, some rural areas have no available broadband service offerings, making it difficult to determine the appropriate discounts under the Primary Program.[415] Second, according to some participants, the flat-rate discount allows Pilot projects to focus on efficiency when designing their networks instead of making sure they take maximum advantage of the urban/rural price differential.[416] Third, the flat-rate discount allows USAC to process application forms more efficiently because it does not require the use of complicated formulas based on mileage-based support or the urban/rural price differential to determine discount levels.[417] The flat-rate discount provides predictability to the funding amounts projects can expect to receive.[418]

103.   The flat-rate discount also makes it easier for USAC to fund Pilot projects' shared services and backbone connections. The Pilot Program requires consortium participants to submit a detailed line-item cost worksheet that includes a breakdown of total network costs when submitting their funding requests to USAC ("Network Cost Worksheet"). According to USAC, shared services and backbone connections are much easier to fund via the Network Cost Worksheet because eligible services are funded at a flat-rate discount level, without regard to mileage or to comparisons between urban and rural rates, as would be required under the Primary Program.[419]

I.   Discount Percentage

104.   A number of Pilot projects state that the size of the discount (85 percent) was a key reason for their success in attracting HCPs to join their networks and start telemedicine programs.[420] Some stated that the 85 percent discount makes broadband affordable for many HCPs.[421] By contrast, the

---

[413] See USAC Observations Letter at 6-7; NRHA Dec. 21 Ex Parte Letter at 1 (some health care providers do not apply for the Primary Program due to uncertainty as to how much of a discount they may receive).

[414] USAC Observations Letter at 7. See supra n. 411.

[415] See Pilot Conference Call Mar. 13 Ex Parte Letter (PMHA et al.) at 3; Pilot Conference Call Mar. 16 Ex Parte Letter (ARCHIE et al.) at 3.

[416] See USAC Observations Letter at 5.

[417] See USAC Observations Letter at 7. See also Pilot Conference Call Mar. 26 Ex Parte Letter (WNYRAHEC et al.) at 4 (Pilot projects discussing the simplicity of the flat rate discount as compared to the urban/rural differential in the Primary Program).

[418] See Pilot Conference Call Mar. 13 Ex Parte Letter (PMHA et al.) at 3; PSPN Feb. 23 Ex Parte Letter at 2.

[419] See USAC Observations Letter at 4, 6-7; USAC May 4 Data Letter at 4.

[420] See Colorado Feb. 28 Ex Parte Letter at 2; Cabarrus Health Alliance et al. Comments at 1; Letter from Frank J. Trembulak, Executive Vice President, Chief Operating Officer, Geisinger Health System, to Marlene H. Dortch, Secretary, Federal Communications Commission, WC Docket No. 02-60 at 2 (filed April 4, 2012).

[421] See Colorado Feb. 28 Ex Parte Letter at 2; PSPN Feb. 23 Ex Parte Letter at 2; Pilot Conference Call Mar. 13 Ex Parte Letter (PMHA et al.) at 3.

urban/rural price differential in the Primary Program does not offer the same level of discount across the board.[422]

105.   As discussed above in Section III.H, some projects note that the 85 percent discount enables projects to provide higher bandwidths to health care providers in their networks at nearly the same, if not lower, prices than they were paying for lower bandwidth services. Additionally, some projects report that the 85 percent discount encourages urban health care providers to engage and participate in their networks.[423] Some projects observe that the 85 percent discount is large enough to encourage the use of broadband connections for telemedicine programs.[424]

106.   Most projects were able to find funding for the program-required 15 percent match, although even this amount was challenging for some HCPs.[425] Several projects state that the highest matching requirement they could support was 25-30 percent of the entire project (i.e., 70-75 percent discount level).[426] In the majority of Pilot projects, participating health care providers themselves provide funds for the minimum 15 percent contribution to network costs.[427] Over 50 percent of Pilot projects report that they look solely to their participating health care providers for the 15 percent matching funds,[428] while nearly 20 percent rely on participating health care provider funds in conjunction

[422] For example, USAC found that eligible funding percentages for HCPs under the Primary Program would have ranged between 51.04% and 89.79% (excluding Alaska). USAC Observations Letter at 6. See also Pilot Conference Call Mar. 13 Ex Parte Letter (PMHA et al.) at 3.

[423] Pilot Conference Call Mar. 13 Ex Parte Letter (PMHA et al.) at 3; Colorado Feb. 28 Ex Parte Letter at 2 (85 percent discount provided sites with incentive to collaborate in a network instead of acting alone).

[424] See, e.g., Letter from Frank J. Trembulak, Executive Vice President, Chief Operating Officer, Geisinger Health System, to Marlene H. Dortch, Secretary, Federal Communications Commission, WC Docket No. 02-60, at 2 (filed April 4, 2012) (noting that 85 percent discount level lowered one barrier to participation in telemedicine programs), Colorado Feb. 28 Ex Parte Letter at 2 (explaining that this degree of subsidy allowed sites that had formerly done without broadband or were using substandard services (by health care information exchange standards) to "fully participate at bandwidth speeds necessary for telemedicine applications").

[425] See Pilot Conference Call Mar. 13 Ex Parte Letter (PMHA et al.) at 2; Pilot Conference Call Mar. 16 Ex Parte Letter (ARCHIE et al.) at 1; Pilot Conference Call Mar. 26 Ex Parte Letter (AEN et al.) at 1.

[426] Pilot Conference Call Mar. 13 Ex Parte Letter (PMHA et al.) at 3.

[427] Based on staff review of Pilot participant 2011-2012 quarterly reports.

[428] Quarterly Report of Bacon County Health Services, Inc., WC Docket No. 02-60, at 10 (filed Jan. 26, 2012); Quarterly Report of Colorado Health Care Connections, WC Docket No. 02-60, at 8 (filed Jan. 27, 2012); Quarterly Report of Communicare, WC Docket No. 02-60, at 3 (filed Jan. 30, 2012); Quarterly Report of Frontier Access to Rural Healthcare in Montana, WC Docket No. 02-60, at 11 (filed Jan. 12, 2012); Quarterly Report of Heartland Unified Broadband Network (HUBNet), WC Docket No. 02-60, at 55 (filed Jan. 30, 2012); Quarterly Report of Indiana Telehealth Network, WC Docket No. 02-60, at 34 (filed Jan. 27, 2012); Quarterly Report of Iowa Rural Health Telecommunications Program, WC Docket No. 02-60, at 26 (filed Jan. 13, 2012); Quarterly Report of Kentucky Behavioral Telehealth Network, WC Docket No. 02-60, at 30 (filed Jan. 27, 2012); Quarterly Report of New England Telehealth Consortium, WC Docket No. 02-60, at 81 (filed Jan. 27, 2012); Quarterly Report of North Country Telemedicine Project, WC Docket No. 02-60, at 17 (filed Jan. 30, 2012); Quarterly Report of Northeast Ohio Regional Health Information Organization, WC Docket No. 02-60, at 22 (filed Jan. 30, 2012); Quarterly Report of Pacific Broadband Telehealth Demonstration Project (PBTD), WC Docket No. 02-60, at 14-15 (filed Jan. 29, 2012); Quarterly Report of Pathways Community Behavioral Healthcare, WC Docket No. 02-60, at 13 (filed Jan. 30, 2012); Quarterly Report of Pennsylvania Mountains Healthcare Alliance, WC Docket No. 02-60, at 9 (filed Feb. 6, 2012); Quarterly Report of Rocky Mountain HealthNet, WC Docket No. 02-60, at 7, 10 (filed Jan. 27, 2012); Quarterly Report of Rural Wisconsin Healthcare Cooperative Information Technology Network, WC Docket No. 02-60, at 22 (filed Jan. 31, 2012); Quarterly Report of Sanford Health Collaboration and Communication Channel, WC Docket No. 02-60, at 4-5 (filed Jan. 30, 2012); Quarterly Report of Southern Ohio Healthcare Network, WC

(continued . . .)

with state and/or federal grants.[429] Within a Pilot project, costs per participant are often allocated based on the amount of bandwidth the provider has purchased.[430] Two Pilot projects noted that excess capacity agreements have proved to be an important revenue stream to offset not only the 15 percent contribution, but also to ensure the network achieves long term sustainability.[431] The figure below lists the sources of the 15 percent contribution relied upon by Pilot projects, as reported to the Commission. The sustainability plans submitted by projects show sources of ongoing support after expiration of Pilot Program funding, as discussed above in Section V.F.

Figure 20 – Source of 15% Match[432]

Source of 15% Match	Count	Percentage
Participants	27	52%
Participants; State Grant and/or Federal Grant	12	24%
Project Coordinator	5	10%
No response	2	4%
State Grant	1	2%
Participants; State Grant; Private Grant	1	2%
Private Grant	1	2%
Participants; Excess Capacity	1	2%
Excess Capacity	1	2%
Total	*50*	*100%*

107. Of the projects that rely upon participating members for matching funds, many also ask their members to help support ongoing network system operation and maintenance costs. While some projects require participants to adjust operating budgets to accommodate operation and maintenance costs, others projects include such costs in participant membership or connectivity fees. For example,

(. . . continued from previous page) ———————————————

Docket No. 02-60, at 10-11 (filed Jan. 30, 2012) (also received loan); Quarterly Report of Southwest Telehealth Access Grid (SWTAG), WC Docket No. 02-60, at 11 (filed Jan. 27, 2012); Quarterly Report of St. Joseph's Hospital, WC Docket No. 02-60, at 6 (filed Jan. 20, 2012); Quarterly Report of Southwest Alabama Mental Health Consortium, WC Docket No. 02-60, at 7 (filed Jan. 30, 2012); Quarterly Report of Texas Health Information Network Collaborative, WC Docket No. 02-60, at 3-4 (filed Jan. 30, 2012); Quarterly Report of Virginia Acute Stroke Telehealth Project (VAST), Docket No. 02-60, at 5 (filed Jan. 30, 2012); Quarterly Report of Western New York Rural Area Health Education Center, WC Docket No. 02-60, at 15 (filed Oct. 26, 2011).

[429] Quarterly Report of Adirondack Champlain Telemedicine Information Network (ACTION), WC Docket No. 02-60, at 5 (filed Jan. 20, 2012); Quarterly Report of Erlanger, WC Docket No. 02-60, at 5-6 (filed Jan. 30, 2012); Quarterly Report of Illinois Rural HealthNet Consortium, WC Docket No. 02-60, at 14-15 (filed Jan. 24, 2012); Quarterly Report of Michigan Public Health Institute, WC Docket No. 02-60, at 17 (filed Jan. 30, 2012); Quarterly Report of Oregon Health Network, WC Docket No. 02-60, at 6 (filed Jan. 31, 2012); Quarterly Report of Palmetto State Providers Network, WC Docket No. 02-60, at 42 (filed Jan. 30, 2012); Quarterly Report of Tennessee Telehealth Network, WC Docket No. 02-60, at 7 (filed Jan. 31, 2012); Quarterly Report of Utah Telehealth Network, WC Docket No. 02-60, at 6 (filed Jan. 30, 2012); Quarterly Report of West Virginia Telehealth Alliance, WC Docket No. 02-60, at 11 (filed Jan. 30, 2012).

[430] *See* Quarterly Report of Adirondack Champlain Telemedicine Information Network (ACTION), WC Docket No. 02-60, at 11 (filed Jan. 20, 2012) ("eligible participants will pay 15% of the network service delivery costs for each site connection, based on the amount of bandwidth they choose to purchase"); Quarterly Report of Bacon County Health Service, WC Docket No. 02-60, at 10 (filed Jan. 26, 2012) ("costs are allocated among HCPs based on the contracted connectivity and equipment specified for each individual HCP site").

[431] Quarterly Report of Health Information Exchange of Montana, WC Docket No. 02-60, at 9 (filed Jan. 24, 2012); Rural Nebraska Healthcare Network, WC Docket No. 02-60, at 8 (filed Jan. 26, 2012).

[432] Based on staff review of Pilot participant 2011-2012 quarterly reports.

the Utah Telehealth Network participants' monthly membership fees include not only the network costs of a T-1 line, but also technical support services and videoconferencing fees.[433] By comparison, St. Joseph's Hospital requires consortium members to budget for maintenance and other recurring expenses through "each facility's normal operation budget process."[434]

VI.   CONCLUSION

108.   The universal service support provided through the Pilot Program has done much to foster the creation and extension of broadband networks of health care providers throughout the country. The Pilot projects successfully demonstrate the value of broadband connectivity among rural and urban health care providers. They offer numerous examples of how telemedicine and other telehealth applications provided over broadband can produce better quality health care for patients in rural areas, better access to medical specialists, and lower health care costs.

109.   Fifty Pilot projects are active in 38 states, and many are state-wide or regional networks. Most are well on the way to full implementation. The flexibility in the Program's design produced a wide range among the projects in size, geographic coverage, network configurations, and features. Many included a type of hub-and-spoke design, connecting rural health care providers to larger health care providers that are often located in urban areas. Although the Pilot Program provides support for both network construction and purchased services, the majority of Pilot projects have chosen to purchase services from third-party providers, and many have taken advantage of longer term leasing arrangements to obtain the bandwidth and quality they need.

110.   The Pilot Program also demonstrates the cost savings, relative administrative simplicity, and network-facilitating value of a consortium approach. When coupled with competitive bidding and multi-year funding, the consortium approach also has the potential to yield higher bandwidth, lower prices, and better service quality for participating health care providers. Allowing urban health care providers to participate in the program also has yielded many benefits. In many projects, the urban HCPs were project leaders, contributed administrative and technical resources, and provided access to medical specialists through telemedicine.

111.   The data and observations set forth in this Staff Report should provide valuable to the Commission as it moves forward on reform of its permanent Rural Health Care program, enabling the Commission to take full advantage of the opportunity to learn from the valuable experience of fifty different Pilot projects.

---

[433] Quarterly Report of Utah Telehealth Network, WC Docket No. 02-60, at 13 (filed Jan. 30, 2012).

[434] Quarterly Report of St. Joseph's Hospital, WC Docket No. 02-60, at 7 (filed Jan. 20, 2012).

APPENDIX A
STATUS OF PILOT PROJECTS BY STATE

LEAD STATE (Other States)	PROJECT	STATUS
AK	**Alaska eHealth Network**	**Active**
AL	Alabama Pediatric Health Access Network	Withdrew
AL	**Southwest Alabama Mental Health Consortium**	**Active**
AL	**Northwest Alabama Mental Health Center**	**Active**
AL	Rural Healthcare Consortium of Alabama	Withdrew
AR	**Arkansas Telehealth Network**	**Active**
AZ	**Arizona Rural Community Health Information Exchange**	**Active**
AZ	Tohono O'odham Nation Department of Information Technology	Missed 6/30/11 deadline
CA	**California Telehealth Network**	**Active**
CO	**Colorado Health Care Connections**	**Active**
CO	**Rocky Mountain HealthNet**	**Active**
FL	Big Bend Regional Healthcare Information Organization	Missed 6/30/11 deadline
GA	**Bacon County Health Services, Inc.**	**Active**
HI (GU, AS, MP)	**Pacific Broadband Telehealth Demonstration Project**	**Active**
IA (IL)	**Iowa Health System**	**Active**
IA (NE, SD)	**Iowa Rural Health Telecommunications Program**	**Active**
IL	**Illinois Rural HealthNet Consortium**	**Active**
IN	**Indiana Telehealth Network**	**Active**
KS	KanEd	Withdrew
KY	DCH Health System	Missed 6/30/11 deadline
KY	**Communicare**	**Active**
KY	**Kentucky Behavioral Telehealth Network**	**Active**
LA	**Louisiana Department of Hospitals**	**Active**
ME	**Rural Western and Central Maine Broadband Initiative**	**Active**
ME (VT, NH)	**New England Telehealth Consortium**	**Active**
MI	**Michigan Public Health Institute**	**Active**
MN	**Greater Minnesota Telehealth Broadband Initiative**	**Active**
MO	**Missouri Telehealth Network**	**Active**
MO	**Pathways Community Behavioral Healthcare, Inc.**	**Active**
MS	University of Mississippi Medical Center	Missed 6/30/11 deadline
MT	**Health Information Exchange of Montana**	**Active**
MT	**Frontier Access to Rural Healthcare in Montana**	**Active**
NC	**North Carolina Telehealth Network**	**Active**
NC	Albemarle Health	Merged[435]
NC	Western Carolina University	Merged[436]
NC	University Health Systems of Eastern Carolina	Merged[437]
ND	Health Care Research & Education Network	Withdrew
NE	**Rural Nebraska Healthcare Network**	**Active**

---

[435] Albemarle Health merged with the North Carolina Telehealth Network. *See Rural Health Care Support Mechanism, North Carolina Telehealth Network, Albemarle Health, Western Carolina University, and University Health Systems of Eastern Carolina Request for Merger of Pilot Program Projects,* WC Docket No. 02-60, Order, DA 09-1696 (Wireline Comp. Bur. rel. July 31, 2009).

[436] Western Carolina University merged with the North Carolina Telehealth Network. *See id.*

[437] University Health Systems of Eastern Carolina merged with the North Carolina Telehealth Network. *See id.*

LEAD STATE (Other States)	PROJECT	STATUS
NM (AZ, TX, CO, CA, NV, UT)	**Southwest Telehealth Access Grid**	Active
NY	**North Country Telemedicine Project**	Active
NY	**Western New York Rural Area Health Education Center**	Active
NY	**Adirondack-Champlain Telemedicine Information Network**	Active
OH	**Northeast Ohio Regional Health Information Organization**	Active
OH	**Southern Ohio Health Care Network**	Active
OH	Holzer Consolidated Health Systems	Merged[438]
OR	**Oregon Health Network**	Active
PA	**Geisinger Health System**	Active
PA	**Northwestern Pennsylvania Telemedicine Initiative**	Active
PA (NY)	**Northeast HealthNet**	Active
PA	**Pennsylvania Mountains Healthcare Alliance**	Active
PA	Penn State Milton S. Hershey Medical Center	Missed 6/30/11 deadline
PA	**Juniata Valley Network**	**Merged[439]**
PR	Puerto Rico Health Department	Missed 6/30/11 deadline
SC	**Palmetto State Providers Network**	Active
SD (ND, IA, MN, NE, WY)	**Heartland Unified Broadband Network**	Active
SD (IA, MN)	**Sanford Health Collaboration and Communication Channel**	Active
TN (VA)	Mountain States Health Alliance	Missed 6/30/11 deadline
TN (GA)	**Erlanger Health System**	Active
TN (KY)	**Tennessee Telehealth Network**	Active
TX	**Texas Health Information Network Collaborative**	Active
TX	Texas Healthcare Network	Merged[440]
UT	**Utah Telehealth Network**	Active
VA	**Virginia Acute Stroke Telehealth Project**	Active
WA	Association of Washington Public Hospital Districts	Missed 6/30/11 deadline
WI	**St. Joseph's Hospital**	Active
WI	**Rural Wisconsin Health Cooperative ITN**	Active
WV	**West Virginia Telehealth Alliance**	Active
WY	**Wyoming Network for Telehealth (WyNETTE)**	Active

---

[438] Holzer Consolidated Health Systems merged with the Southern Ohio Health Care Network. *See Rural Health Care Mechanism, Holzer Consolidated Health Systems and Southern Ohio Health Care Network Request for Merger of Rural Health Care Pilot Program Projects,* WC Docket No. 02-60, Order, 23 FCC Rcd 17396 (Wireline Comp. Bur. 2008).

[439] Juniata Valley Network merged with the Pennsylvania Mountains Healthcare Alliance. *See Rural Health Care Mechanism, Juanita Valley Network and Pennsylvania Mountains Healthcare Alliance Request for Merger of Rural Health Care Pilot Program Projects,* WC Docket No. 02-60, Order, 24 FCC Rcd 10606 (Wireline Comp. Bur. 2009).

[440] Texas Healthcare Network merged with the Texas Health Information Network Collaborative. *See Rural Health Care Support Mechanism, Texas Healthcare Network and Texas Health Information Network Collaborative Request for Merger of Rural Health Care Pilot Program Projects,* WC Docket No. 0-2-60, Order, 24 FCC Rcd 4587 (Wireline Comp. Bur. 2009).

APPENDIX B[441]
PILOT PROJECT DESCRIPTIONS AND GOALS

Project	Project Description	Project Goals
Adirondack-Champlain Telemedicine Information Network (ACTION)	ACTION has leased fiber/Ethernet services that provide the engineering, materials, construction, implementation, maintenance, and sustaining network support for a dedicated, managed router/firewall service over a secure fiber/Ethernet broadband network. The network will provide 100 Mbps and 1 Gbps fiber/Ethernet and will also provide a 500Mb connection to the public Internet as part of this leased service.	Assist regional health care providers to increase access to an information system that will be fully utilized to: <ul><li>Improve patient safety (alert for medication errors, drug allergies, and emergency response);</li><li>Improve health care quality (make available complete electronic medical records, test results and x-rays at the point of care, integrate health information from multiple sources and providers, incorporate the use of decision support tools with guidelines and research results, etc.); and,</li><li>Create a health information system for the purpose of sharing common patient medical information among ACTION members to improve quality of care and maximize cost efficiencies.</li></ul>
Alaska eHealth Network	Comprised primarily of rural health care practitioners, the consortium will unify and increase the capacity of disparate health care networks throughout Alaska in order to connect with urban health centers and access services in the lower 48 states. Approximately 270 facilities will be connected.	Improve broadband performance for 109 Alaskan health care organizations to better facilitate health information exchange, electronic health records (EHR) performance, digital imaging solutions and telemedicine.
Arizona Rural Community Health Information Exchange (ARCHIE)	New telecommunications connectivity for members of a health coalition in a rural county with little existing telecom infrastructure. Once connectivity is established, ARCHIE members plan to create a health information exchange (HIE) to share clinical data across a large geographical area with small population centers. ARCHIE will participate in telemedicine, distance learning, and public health data accumulation as these services become available.	<ul><li>Increase health telecommunications infrastructure in Cochise County, AZ.</li><li>Initiate E-Health data sharing among health providers in Cochise County, with eventual inclusion of all health sectors (pharmacy, EMS, behavioral health).</li><li>Increase health data collection and surveillance utilizing public health systems, disease registries).</li></ul>

[441] USAC May 5 Data Letter at App. A.

Project	Project Description	Project Goals
Arkansas Telehealth Network	Four existing networks will be consolidated and expanded using broadband connections to enable better patient care, including electronic records management, and coordinating responses to major public health incidents.	• Consolidate the state's existing telehealth networks; • Update and expand the statewide network to improve rural access; • Connect to Internet2 and Arkansas' dark fiber backbone, and • Schedule and manage the 24/7 needs of the statewide network through a centralized management system.
Bacon County Health Services, Inc.	A new 1 Gbps network will connect approximately 18 public and non-profit health care facilities in rural and urban locations in Georgia to an existing network, enabling telemedicine services, distance education, research, and effective disaster response.	The goals and purposes of the project are to provide improved health care to area residents, and to provide leadership in the development, coordination and rationalization of health care services.
California Telehealth Network (CTN)	CTN will connect over 800 California health care providers in underserved areas to a state- and nation-wide broadband network dedicated to health care.	CTN's goals are to advance the use of telecommunications and health care technology and to significantly increase access to acute, primary and preventive health care in rural America.
Colorado Health Care Connections (CHCC)	CHCC is a statewide, high speed private broadband network connecting approximately 95 hospitals and clinics enabling telehealth and collaboration between state organizations.	Goals are to grow the network, create partnerships, enable telehealth, and facilitate collaboration.
Communicare	A T1-based network connecting approximately 20 facilities specializing in mental health services will enable video consultation and other videoconferencing applications.	Establish point-to-point broadband links to Communicare service sites for purpose of providing mental health services, including telepsychiatry/therapy.
Erlanger Health System	Erlanger will extend an existing fiber network to deliver patient care, video consultations, and data exchange, to approximately 10 health care facilities serving residents in sparsely populated regions of southeast Tennessee and smaller areas of northern Georgia, and western North Carolina.	Improve rural access to a broader range of health care services.
Frontier Access to Rural Healthcare in Montana (FAhRM)	A state-wide network, using T1 connections to a high speed backbone, will connect approximately 140 health care facilities to provide high definition videoconferencing, maintain electronic health records, and provide other services.	The goal of the FAhRM project is to support the continued development and expansion of a reliable, cost effective telehealth network-of-networks that has sufficient, scalable bandwidth from defined hubs to the cloud to support the increasing demands for the delivery of health care applications in rural areas. The FAhRM pilot project will provide for end to end networks allowing efficient, seamless and dynamic routing of data from and between six hub-site partners to 48 rural spoke-site entities.
Geisinger Health System	Existing network structures covering approximately 15 facilities will be enhanced and connected using high bandwidth connections to transfer radiographs, improve electronic record systems, and enable other telemedicine services.	To install a foundation of high speed bandwidth to multiple rural outlying hospitals then build multiple specialty telemedicine services over that foundation to accommodate rural residents and keep much needed revenue at rural outlying hospitals.

Project	Project Description	Project Goals
Greater Minnesota Telehealth Broadband Initiative	Is an affiliation of several existing health care networks in Minnesota and North Dakota representing over 140 health care facilities that is building a robust, reliable, and secure broadband network utilizing broadband connections up to 1Gbps, MPLS technology, and a Network Operating Center.	• Create a cost effective and medical grade telehealth delivery service infrastructure for both rural and urban health care facilities. • Increase access to health care throughout the state and the region. • Allow for statewide and regional health information exchange. • Promote technical standards and operational best practices to reduce costs, boost performance, and improve ease-of-use of telehealth applications.
Health Information Exchange of Montana	Establish a dedicated, robust fiber optic network with connections to at least twenty-four participating sites to enable distance consultation, electronic record keeping and exchange, disaster readiness, clinical research and distance education services. The new network will also serve as a natural connection point to Internet2, UCAN and the Northern Tier Network.	• Develop a fiber optic network to support electronic health records, health information exchange, remote digital imaging and telemedicine/telehealth. • Provide network connections to support distance learning for health care education programs.
Heartland Unified Broadband Network	Existing networks will interconnect to a fiber-optic network of about 180 facilities with connections to Internet2.	The expanded and enhanced network will address health problems of the area's aging population, increase the use and quality of teleradiology and telehealth activities, and improve distance education programs.
Illinois Rural HealthNet Consortium	This statewide network will serve approximately 87 health care facilities and connect to Internet2. More than 95% of the connected locations will have connectivity at speeds ranging from 100 Mbps to 1 Gbps.	Participating health care providers will be able to meet new HIE and HIT requirements, treat more patients, consult with specialists while the patient is at the hospital, and send and receive radiological and digital imaging expeditiously, such as mammograms and C-scans.
Indiana Telehealth Network	The network will connect approximately 60 rural health care facilities throughout Indiana, including approximately 20 of the 35 critical access hospitals, several rural and urban hospitals, and approximately 30 community mental health centers and rural health clinics providing speeds from 5 mbps to 1 Gbps. The hospitals will serve as capacity hubs connecting to smaller health facilities.	To improve the health and well-being of Indiana residents, particularly those in rural areas, through the utilization of a dedicated broadband health network to deliver telehealth applications including but not limited to telemedicine, health information exchange, distance education and training, public health surveillance, emergency preparedness, and trauma system development.

Project	Project Description	Project Goals
Iowa Health System	The new network connections will link approximately 78 health care facilities, including 52 rural facilities, to an existing statewide, dedicated, broadband health care network and National LambdaRail.	• Enable health-care professionals to deliver better care to their patients. • Whether it is through more effective sharing of medical information, remote radiology, diagnostic services or any other advanced tele-health application accessible over the network, the goal is to provide health-care professionals a capability to deliver better care. • Potentially connect to other regional networks around the country, creating the footprint for a national health-care network capability.
Iowa Rural Health Health Telecommunicat ions Program	To provide last mile fiber connection for participating Iowa, Nebraska and South Dakota hospitals to the closest appropriate ICN Point of Presence (POP) with 1 gigabit Ethernet electronics connection from each hospital to one of 19 ICN aggregation points and using Internet Protocol (IP)/Multiprotocol Label Switching (MPLS) electronics to connect the 19 aggregation points with a resilient (10) gigabit backbone that creates a statewide health care network, service assurance, service level management, and customer reporting functions.	• Solve the problems of isolation, travel and limited resources that constrain health care delivery in rural Iowa by providing increased bandwidth for clinical and administrative applications of the hospital's choosing. • Leverage current proven Iowa Communication Network assets to extend broadband service to rural Iowa hospitals. • Improve access to and availability of clinical and administrative services, data and information.

Project	Project Description	Project Goals
Kentucky Behavioral Telehealth Network	The network will connect community mental health facilities in Appalachian southeastern Kentucky to major urban hospitals to improve patient access to a full range of medical professionals. Approximately 27 facilities will be connected.	• Plan a Kentucky state wide rural health care network that links the existing statewide network of regional behavioral health providers with primary medical care providers and hospitals to improve access to a full range of medical care for persons with co-morbid medical conditions. • Design a Kentucky statewide rural telehealth network that seamlessly interfaces with existing state networks, makes uses of existing capacity, in place resources and technology combined with the best of new technologies using a design team of highly qualified consulting systems and telecommunications engineers. • Establish a statewide telehealth network of behavioral health care providers linking them to each other, primary medical care, and specialty medical care resources that makes use of the national Internet2 network if necessary, when appropriate and available, utilize the Internet2 infrastructure, insuring maximum available bandwidth for the benefit of those rural areas medically underserved. • Implement, train and develop policies, procedures and clinical protocols that guarantee a swift adoption of the new technology as a resource to all members of the provider network. • Develop Implement and plan for network self sufficiency and sustainability.
Louisiana Department of Hospitals	The Department will connect approximately 168 facilities, about 93 of which are rural, to a broadband network that will link public and private health care providers to each other, enable patient access to medical specialists, and provide rapid and coordinated crises responses.	To promote access to telehealth and telemedicine applications.
Michigan Public Health Institute	New network infrastructure will connect Michigan health care providers and health networks to each other and Internet2 at speeds ranging from 1.5 Mbps to 1 Gbps and higher. The network will directly network well over 100 facilities, primarily rural and most located in underserved areas of the state.	• To network eight rural hospitals in the Thumb area of Michigan by building four towers and providing equipment for nine towers, with the system owned by the hospital consortium; • To network 72 health care providers throughout the state (including two hospitals in the eight-hospital Thumb network) via a secure, high-speed, health care-dedicated, MPLS network owned and operated by the vendor; and • To create private fiber networks for four hospital systems (covering a total of 34 sites).

Project	Project Description	Project Goals
Missouri Telehealth Network	The network will create a 2 Gbps statewide dedicated telehealth backbone, enabling new telemedicine services including those requiring high-definition video streaming. The network will also add about 32 facilities to an existing network of approximately 127 facilities and connect to Internet2.	• N/A
New England Telehealth Consortium	A multi-state telehealth network will deliver remote trauma consultation and expansive telemedicine by linking approximately 500 primarily rural health care facilities – including hospitals, behavioral health sites, correctional facility clinics, and community health care centers – in Vermont, New Hampshire and Maine to urban hospitals and universities throughout New England.	The goal of NETC is to augment health care services, health information exchange services, research, and education by enhancing broadband capacity and providing Internet2 services to support existing programs and the implementation of more effective and sustainable telehealth and telemedicine services.
North Carolina Telehealth Network	Regional network will connect approximately 100 health care facilities across North Carolina including public health clinics, free clinics, federally qualified community health centers (FQHCs), and hospitals.	Create and sustain a broadband network for health and care in NC focusing on public and non-profit providers.
North Country Telemedicine Project	A total of 27 health care facilities in a poor, sparsely populated region of northern New York are connected via a leased fiber/Ethernet service that includes a 500Mb connection to the public Internet at speeds ranging from 10 to 100 Mbps. Expected services will include teledermatology, teleradiology, diabetes, CME and telepsychiatry through video conferencing and education. The network serves the region surrounding Fort Drum, home to the most deployed soldiers in the United States Army.	• Identify the health care needs of the community surrounding and including Fort Drum, NY. • Develop a plan to address and support the health care needs of the community utilizing telemedicine and telemedical education. • Foster a platform for the collection and exchange of information to promote health through coordinated, area-wide health services programs.
Northeast HealthNet	The current approved application was for 21 entities of which approximately 75% are connected. This includes a composition of both urban and rural health care settings and provides for the access of diagnostic and clinical information.	The goals of the program are to enhance the current exchange of health care information as well as to further develop clinical education and telehealth initiatives.

Project	Project Description	Project Goals
Northeast Ohio Regional Health Information Organization	The expansion of an existing network to connect approximately 16 medical facilities at speeds ranging from 100 Mbps to 1 Gbps. The expansion is predominantly within the Northeast Ohio geography.	• Make all necessary health care information available to patients and providers where it is needed, when it is needed. • Provide a secure, confidential, patient-controlled environment for health information exchange. • Provide opportunities for patients to more actively participate in their health care. • Reduce duplicative testing, administrative burdens, and other barriers to cost-effective health care. • Enable health care research using de-identified data. • Reduce disparities in health care. • Provide transparency to enhance quality assessment and value comparison. • Enhance the economic viability of the region.
Northwest Alabama Mental Health Center	This broadband network links six community mental health centers with the Walker Baptist Medical Center. Five network sites have 15 Mbps service and two sites have 100 Mbps service.	Project goals are to provide telepsychiatry, VOIP, data and internet services over the broadband network.
Northwestern Pennsylvania Telemedicine Initiative	This project was designed to bring much needed specialty care to rural communities so that travel and time off from work may be minimized. With telemedicine, the community hospitals may be able to stop the migration of many patients (and subsequently revenue) to the larger tertiary care facilities. The technology was also to assist in the recruitment and retention of physicians for the rural communities.	• To improve access to a broad range of nationally recognized medical specialty services and help provide standardization of care for patients. • To encourage physicians, nurse, and allied health professionals to establish practices and services and remain in the rural communities • To increase public safety and promote the cooperation of smaller community hospitals to share services.
Oregon Health Network (OHN)	The network is a "hub & spoke" model that requires all approved telecommunications vendors to peer at a central exchange point (Northwest Access Exchange), and who agree to live up to OHN's strict service level agreements (SLA's). OHN's network configuration and SLAs provide the connectivity infrastructure required to support current and future health care applications that serve the next generation of patient-centered care and health care education.	• Build the core network infrastructure and participant base footprint necessary to build the value and momentum needed to support a sustainable statewide health care network. • Provide as much middle-mile infrastructure as possible throughout Oregon to eventually drop the barrier to entry (cost) for the expanded health care community to join the OHN. In addition this infrastructure allows all Oregonians potential access to broadband including schools and business fostering economic growth. • Ensure that all our participants are effectively using OHN to serve the Triple Aim goals of Centers for Medicare & Medicaid Services (CMS).

Project	Project Description	Project Goals
Pacific Broadband Telehealth Demonstration Project	Project will link approximately 96 health care facilities throughout Hawaii and the Pacific Island region to serve a population that spans 11 islands.	• To interconnect health care organizations throughout the State of Hawaii and the Pacific Islands region to a broadband telehealth network that will enable clinicians and support staff to improve the delivery of health care services to rural, remote, and underserved populations. • The network will facilitate many telehealth, telemedicine, clinical, and health related education and training services, and expand the network of service providers through the Internet2.
Palmetto State Providers Network	Connects four rural and underserved regions to a fiber optic backbone being developed in the state and Internet2. FQHC providers will also be added to the network. Network will connect approximately 58 facilities at speeds ranging from 10 Mbps to 10 Gbps.	• Connect all RHC eligible hospitals, clinics and health care providers throughout the state. • Provide a high quality, high speed, fully redundant network to the HCPs of the state. • Provide health care support to underserved areas with specific emphasis on rural counties. • Support telemedicine, telehealth and Health Information Exchange needs for all participants.
Pathways Community Behavioral Healthcare, Inc.	Not-for-profit community mental health center will connect approximately 15 outlying offices to its headquarters. The dedicated T1 network will extend outreach to the current population served, and reduce the costs of recruiting physicians to relocate in rural areas.	To provide clinical and psychiatric care to the rural areas in the state of Missouri.
Pennsylvania Mountains Healthcare Alliance	New broadband network proposed by a consortium of approximately 21 hospitals in rural central and western Pennsylvania will provide a variety of telemedicine services, telehealth services, shared HCIS, and health care information exchange in more than 20 counties. Network will provide a minimum of 10 Mbps service.	Facilitate: • Acquisition of bulk Internet services for hospitals and clinics; • Health information exchange for rural hospitals and clinics; • Telemedicine, telehealth and other shared resources for back office integration; • Shared health care information system implementations reducing cost for critical access hospitals.
Rocky Mountain HealthNet	Statewide, high speed private broadband network connecting approximately 105 mental health centers enabling telehealth and collaboration between state organizations.	Goals are to grow the network, create partnerships, enable telehealth, and facilitate collaboration.
Rural Nebraska Healthcare Network	Consortium of nine rural hospitals and related clinics will upgrade a patchwork of T-1 lines with an advanced fiber network. Network will provide speeds of up to 2 Gbps for a variety of telehealth and telemedicine services in an underserved rural area.	• Improve quality of care and patient safety; • Enable the exchange of health information; • Promote the vision of a system of care for Western Nebraska; • Integrate electronic medical records with other systems; • Expand the use of telehealth and telemedicine.

Project	Project Description	Project Goals
Rural Western and Central Maine Broadband Initiative	New, high-speed fiber optic cable network will serve approximately 80 health care facilities.	To provide broadband access to underserved health care facilities in Central and Western Maine.
Rural Wisconsin Health Cooperative ITN (RWHC ITN)	Will augment an existing shared electronic health records project by providing network management/systems and redundant connectivity from participating hospitals to 2 consortium datacenters, as well as higher speeds that will range from 20 to 100 Mbps.	• Provide high speed, redundant WAN connectivity for facilities and clinics participating in a RWHC ITN Shared EHR Initiative; • To provide redundant connectivity between the redundant hospital-consortium data centers; and • To implement WAN management and security features to maximize uptime.
Sanford Health Collaboration and Communication Channel	Project will connect seven existing networks at speeds of up to 100 Mbps to access administrative services and connect with educational institutions. Facilities served include the Aberdeen, S.D. area Indian Health Services.	• Increase bandwidth to our locations that need increased bandwidth; • Increase failover technology for our locations; • Improve network design.
Southern Ohio Health Care Network	Project will provide approximately 60 facilities with next-generation telemedicine, education, and interconnection with statewide emergency networks and Internet2 by building or purchasing fiber optic rings covering 315 miles. Will also provide connectivity to facilities outside the reach of the fiber optic rings.	To provide approximately 120 health care facilities in 13 counties with next-generation telemedicine, education, and interconnection with statewide emergency networks and Internet2.
Southwest Alabama Mental Health Consortium	Network will connect with Internet2 and provide voice, video and data transmission capabilities to approximately 31 mental health facilities serving 16 counties. Connection speeds range from 3 to 100 Mbps.	N/A
Southwest Telehealth Access Grid	This collaboration of several health care organizations being lead by the UNM CfTH, includes UNM Hospital and Health Sciences Center, Presbyterian Health Systems, Primary Care Association, San Juan Regional Medical Center, Carlsbad Behavioral Health Services, the Albuquerque Area Indian Health Services, and stakeholders in the Navajo Nation; Ft. Defiance, Winslow, and Hardrock service units. Other participants include LCF Research and the Arizona Telemedicine Program. This enhanced broadband network will link hundreds of health care sites and provide the critical infrastructure to support access to telemedicine services, health education, training, research and health information exchange.	Create a network of networks that provides sustainable, affordable broadband that supports health care; telemedicine, eHealth, in order to improve access to health care services, improve health outcomes, and reduce costs in our region and across the nation.

Project	Project Description	Project Goals
St. Joseph's Hospital	St. Joseph's Hospital RHCPP consortium is building a broadband network in Western Wisconsin with to enable a streamlined delivery of telehealth services between providers. Project will link two existing fiber systems in the city of Chippewa Falls to the hospital, two other telehealth facilities and Internet2 in order to expand telemedicine offerings.	• Increase access to health services in rural and underserved communities. • Improve the health care services in the area by providing timely access to health care specialists through the use of telehealth services by linking urban health care providers with rural hospitals.
Tennessee Telehealth Network	Will build on and expand the existing Tennessee Information Infrastructure to serve approximately 450 facilities. Connects to Internet2; will support diabetes research involving three state research centers.	Develop a robust telehealth network throughout the state of Tennessee.
Texas Health Information Network Collaborative	Will expand and improve an existing network serving approximately 40 primarily rural health care facilities at speeds of at least 45 Mbps.	• Provide an interoperable, secure, scalable and cost effective medical grade broadband network to health care facilities in order to connect rural health providers to urban and regional centers so that they may expand health care access, improved services, health information exchange and other services across the entire state of Texas. • Future goals include allowing physicians and health care consumers use the network to collect health information in the home and wherever the patient may be.
Utah Telehealth Network	The project will upgrade and expand an existing network to serve hospitals, clinics, FQHCs, and public health departments throughout Utah. The network will utilize dedicated Ethernet via fiber optics and microwave to provide high speed broadband and improve network reliability. Originally entitled the Utah ARCHES Project, the purpose of the project remains to Advance Rural Connections for Healthcare and E-health Services.	• The expansion of telehealth and telemedicine; • Adoption of health information technology and health information exchange; • Foster collaboration to improve patient care; • Improve training and education for health care professionals.
Virginia Acute Stroke Telehealth Project	Further the deployment of broadband in support of a tele-stroke project. Emphasis is on underserved areas where broadband is lacking (Eastern Shore and the Northern Neck, Middle Peninsula) and those areas that have a strong desire for a tele-stroke project.	Maximize use of FCC Pilot Program funding to bring broadband communications to rural and under served areas of the Commonwealth.
West Virginia Telehealth Alliance	Statewide network will connect approximately 450 facilities to improve connectivity for rural health centers. Project is focused on regions of the state with historically high concentrations of poor and elderly individuals suffering from chronic medical conditions. Will connect to Internet2; speeds range from T1 lines at 1.5 Mbps to 1 Gbps fiber.	• To complete bandwidth upgrades; • Provide guidance to network participants in furthering their Telehealth IQ and assist them to meet each organization's goals by being a conduit of information to those ends.

Project	Project Description	Project Goals
Western New York Rural Area Health Education Center	Network will connect about 40 facilities in rural and urban areas with varying speeds from 10 - 800 Mbps based on facility need in order to provide access to experienced specialty physicians and critical life-saving treatments.	• Creating regional telehealth network; • Provide high speed internet connections at an affordable cost; • Providing health care and health care education on dedicated broadband network; • Connecting those who have with those who need.
Wyoming Network for Telehealth (WyNETTE)	Will help alleviate Wyoming's severe shortage of health care providers and reduce the need for the state's significant rural population to drive long distances for health care by connecting 37 hospitals, primary care clinics, community mental health centers and substance abuse centers. Connects with Internet2.	• Provide high-speed connectivity to participating sites using existing copper connections. • Encourage use of telecommunications to support collaboration among health care providers in Wyoming.

APPENDIX C
PILOT PROJECT COMPOSITION BY HCP TYPE[442]

Project Name	Community / Migrant Health Center	Community Mental Health Center	Local Health Department or Agency	Not-For-Profit Hospital / Dedicated ER of Rural, For-Profit Hospital	Rural Health Clinic or Urban Equivalent	Teaching Hospital, Medical School, Post-Secondary Institution
Adirondack-Champlain Telemedicine Information Network	4			11	33	
Alaska eHealth Network						
Arizona Rural Community Health Information Exchange	1			2	1	
Arkansas Telehealth Network				1		
Bacon County Health Services, Inc.				14	4	
California Telehealth Network	75			26	59	1
Colorado Health Care Connections	31			50	9	
Communicare		8				
Erlanger Health System				9		
Frontier Access to Rural Healthcare in Montana (FAhRM)	1	1		39	6	
Geisinger Health System				7	20	
Greater Minnesota Telehealth Broadband Initiative		10		5		1
Health Information Exchange of Montana	1			10	6	2
Heartland Unified Broadband Network	10	2		35	24	
Illinois Rural HealthNet Consortium		12		66	16	
Indiana Telehealth Network	6	9		27	5	
Iowa Health System	3	2		26	61	
Iowa Rural Health Telecommunications Program				88		

---

[442] USAC Aug. 9 Data Letter at App. G (explaining that the composition of the Alaska eHealth Network and New England Telehealth Consortium are not fully reflected because as of Jan. 31, 2012, they only had funding commitments for network design studies, which were allocated to "Consortium of the Above" and not included in the table).

Project Name	Community / Migrant Health Center	Community Mental Health Center	Local Health Department or Agency	Not-For-Profit Hospital / Dedicated ER of Rural, For-Profit Hospital	Rural Health Clinic or Urban Equivalent	Teaching Hospital, Medical School, Post-Secondary Institution
Kentucky Behavioral Telehealth Network		1				
Louisiana Department of Hospitals			1			
Michigan Public Health Institute	27	8	9	25	14	
Missouri Telehealth Network	26	16		35	17	
New England Telehealth Consortium						
North Carolina Telehealth Network	3		52	23	3	
North Country Telemedicine Project	6	4	2	12	4	
Northeast HealthNet				4	18	
Northeast Ohio Regional Health Information Organization				16		
Northwest Alabama Mental Health Center		6		1		
Northwestern Pennsylvania Telemedicine Initiative				4	3	
Oregon Health Network	8	17		35	82	14
Pacific Broadband Telehealth Demonstration Project				7	8	
Palmetto State Providers Network		39		46	65	5
Pathways Community Behavioral Healthcare, Inc.		16		2		
Pennsylvania Mountains Healthcare Alliance				19		
Rocky Mountain HealthNet		102		1		
Rural Nebraska Healthcare Network	5			10	22	
Rural Western and Central Maine Broadband Initiative	2			4	3	
Rural Wisconsin Health Cooperative ITN				4	2	
Sanford Health Collaboration and Communication Channel				13	21	

Project Name	Community / Migrant Health Center	Community Mental Health Center	Local Health Department or Agency	Not-For-Profit Hospital / Dedicated ER of Rural, For-Profit Hospital	Rural Health Clinic or Urban Equivalent	Teaching Hospital, Medical School, Post-Secondary Institution
Southern Ohio Healthcare Network	17	25	11	18	16	
Southwest Alabama Mental Health Consortium		23				
Southwest Telehealth Access Grid				6	5	
St. Joseph's Hospital				4		
Tennessee Telehealth Network	3				1	
Texas Health Information Network Collaborative				1		
Utah Telehealth Network	11		14	16	11	1
Virginia Acute Stroke Telehealth Project		1				
West Virginia Telehealth Alliance	59			31	2	3
Western New York Rural Area Health Education Center	11			23	2	
Wyoming Network for Telehealth (WyNETTE)		16		16	4	1

APPENDIX D
LIST OF WINNING VENDORS*

Access Integration Specialists
A-D Technologies - Duraline DBA or Arnco Corporation FKA
ADVA Optical Networking NA, Inc. - ADVA Optical Networking
Alamon Telco, Inc.
Alcatel-Lucent USA, Inc
Alexander Open Systems, Inc.
Allo Communications LLC
Alma Telephone Company, Inc.
Alpine Communications, LC
AT&T Corp.
BellSouth Telecommunications, LLC
Blackfoot Communications, Inc.
BNSF Railway Company
Brainstorm Internet, Inc.
Bresnan Communications, LLC - dba Optimum West
BT Conferencing Video Inc
CCI Systems, Inc.
CDW Government, LLC
CenturyLink
Charter Communications - Charter Business and Charter Fiberlink
Ciena Corporation
Citizens Mutual Telephone Company
Citizens Telecomm Co. Of Utah dba Frontier
CoastCom, Inc
Comcast Business Communications
Communication Innovators Inc.
Communication Technologies, Inc.
Conterra Ultra Broadband, LLC
Cox Communications Hampton Roads, LLC
CTSI, LLC, dba Frontier Communications, CTSI Company
Cyan Optics
Development Authority of the North Country
Digicorp, Inc.
Douglas Services Inc
Eastern Oregon Telecom, LLC
Easy Street Online Services, Inc.
EDI, Ltd
Electric Power Board of Chattanooga
Enventis Telecom, Inc.
FiberNet, LLC
Flathead Electric Cooperative, Inc.
FRC, LLC
Frontier Communications of Minnesota, Inc.

Frontier Telenet
Frontier West Virginia Inc.
Fujitsu Network Communications, Inc.
G4S Technology, LLC - Adesta, LLC
GCI Communication Corp
GNJ Construction LLC
Great Basin Electronics, Inc. - Great Basin Electronics
Great Lakes Comnet, Inc.
Gudenkauf Corporation
Hancock Rural Telephone Corporation - DBA NineStar Connect
Hawaiian Telcom, Inc.
Hospers Telephone Exchange Inc. - HTC Communications
iConnects Montana LLC
Illinois Century Network - Central Management Services
Illinois Municipal Broadband Communications Association
Indiana Fiber Network LLC
Information Transport Solutions, Inc.
Inland Development Corporation
INOC, LLC
Integra Telecom of Oregon, Inc.
INX Inc.
Knology of the Black Hills, LLC
Last Mile Inc - Sting Communications
Lightspeed Networks
Long Lines Metro, LLC
Lumos Networks of West Virginia Inc
MapleNet Wireless, Inc.
MasTec North America
MCC Telephony, LLC
McLeodUSA Telecommunications. - DBA PAETEC Business Services
MCNC
Midcontinent Communications
Miles Communications, Inc. - dba Enhanced Telecommunications Corp.
Multilink, Inc.
Muscatine Power & Water
Mutual Telephone Company - Premier Communications
Northern Illinois University
OFS Fitel, LLC
OneCommunity
Pacific Lightnet, Inc. - Wavecom Solutions

PAETEC Communications, Inc.
Peninsula Fiber Network LLC
PenTeleData Limited Partnership I
Perry-Spencer Rural Tel Coop Inc - dba PSC
Professional Information Networks - ProInfoNet
Pulaski White Rural Telephone Cooperative,
Incor
Quantum Communications, LLC
Rochester Telephone Co., Inc.
Ronan Telephone Company
Rural Wisconsin Health Cooperative
Saint Vincent Health Center - SVHC
Information Technology Network Services
Sho-Me Technologies, LLC
Sjoberg's, Inc. - Sjoberg's Cable TV, Inc
Smithville Digital, LLC
Sorrento Networks, Inc.
South Dakota Network, LLC - DBA's-SDN
Communications SDN Technologies
Southwestern Bell Telephone Company - AT&T
Southwest
Spencer Municipal Communications Utility
State of Iowa, Iowa Telecommunication &

Technology - Iowa Communications Network
Texcel Inc.
The Chillicothe Telephone Company - Horizon
Chillicothe Telephone Company
Thumb Radio Inc
Time Warner Cable Information Services
Tribal One Broadband Technologies, LLC -
ORCA Communications
TriLightNET LLC
University Corporation for Advanced Internet
Development - Internet2
Verizon Network Integration Corp.
Vision Net, Inc - Montana Advanced
Information Network, Inc.
West Alabama T.V. Cable Company Inc
Westelcom Networks Inc
Western Fibernet, LLC
Windstream Communications, Inc.
WiscNet
Wisconsin Bell, Inc. - AT&T Wisconsin
Zayo Enterprise Networks LLC - ZEN
Zito Media Voice, LLC

* Source: USAC May 4 USAC Data Letter, App. C.

APPENDIX E
LIST OF *EX PARTE* FILINGS AND CITATIONS

PARTY	ABBREVIA TION	DATE OF FILING	SHORT CITE	FULL CITE
Universal Service Administrative Company	USAC	Feb. 23, 2010	USAC Feb. 23 Letter	Letter from William England, Vice President, Rural Health Care Division, USAC, to Marlene H. Dortch, Secretary, Federal Communications Commission, WC Docket No. 02-60 (filed Feb. 23, 2010) (USAC Feb. 23 Letter).
Health Information Exchange of Montana	HIEM	Sept. 22, 2010	HIEM Sept. 22 *Ex Parte* Letter	Letter from David LaFuria, Counsel for Health Information Exchange of Montana, to Marlene H. Dortch, Secretary, WC Docket No. 02-60 (Sept. 22, 2010) (HIEM Sept. 22 *Ex Parte* Letter).
National Rural Health Association	NRHA	Dec. 21, 2011	NRHA Dec. 21 *Ex Parte* Letter	Letter from Christianna Lewis Barnhart, Attorney Advisor, Federal Communications Commission, to Marlene H. Dortch, Secretary, Federal Communications Commission, WC Docket No. 02-60 (filed Dec. 21, 2011) (NRHA Dec. 21 *Ex Parte* Letter).
National Rural Health Resource Center	NRHRC	Dec. 27, 2011	NRHRC Dec. 27 *Ex Parte* Letter	Letter from Chin Yoo, Attorney Advisor, Federal Communications Commission, to Marlene H. Dortch, Secretary, Federal Communications Commission, WC Docket No. 02-60 (filed Dec. 27, 2011) (NRHRC Dec. 27 *Ex Parte* Letter).
U.S. Department of Health Information Services, Office of the National Coordinator for Health Information Technology	ONC	Jan. 6, 2012	ONC Jan. 6 *Ex Parte* Letter	Letter from Linda L. Oliver, Attorney Advisor, Federal Communications Commission, to Marlene H. Dortch, Secretary, Federal Communications Commission, WC Docket No. 02-60 (filed Jan. 6, 2012) (ONC Jan. 6 *Ex Parte* Letter).

PARTY	ABBREVIATION	DATE OF FILING	SHORT CITE	FULL CITE
U.S. Department of Health Information Services, Office of the National Coordinator for Health Information Technology, and Hank Fanberg of CHRISTUS Health	ONC	Jan. 17, 2012	ONC Jan. 17 *Ex Parte* Letter	Letter from Linda L. Oliver, Attorney Advisor, Federal Communications Commission, to Marlene H. Dortch, Secretary, Federal Communications Commission, WC Docket No. 02-60 (filed Jan. 17, 2012) (ONC Jan. 17 *Ex Parte* Letter).
Palmetto State Providers Network	PSPN	Jan. 31, 2012	PSPN Jan. 31 *Ex Parte* Letter	Letter from Jeffrey Mitchell, Counsel for FRC, LLC, on behalf of FRC and PSPN, to Marlene Dortch, Secretary, FCC, WC Docket No. 02-60 (filed Jan. 31, 2012) (PSPN Jan. 31 *Ex Parte* Letter).
Universal Service Administrative Company	USAC	Feb. 17, 2012	USAC Feb. 17 Letter	Letter from Craig Davis, Vice President of Rural Health Care, USAC, to Sharon Gillett, Chief, WCB, WC Docket No. 02-60 (filed February 17, 2012) (USAC Feb. 17 Letter).
Palmetto State Providers Network	PSPN	Feb. 23, 2012	PSPN Feb. 23 *Ex Parte* Letter	Letter from W. Roger Poston II, Palmetto State Providers Network, to Christianna Lewis Barnhart, Attorney Advisor, Federal Communications Commission, WC Docket No. 02-60 (filed Feb. 23, 2012) (PSPN Feb. 23 *Ex Parte* Letter).
Oregon Health Network	OHN	Feb. 28, 2012	OHN Feb. 28 *Ex Parte* Letter	Letter from Kim Klupenger *et al.*, Oregon Health Network, Christianna Lewis Barnhart, Attorney Advisor, Federal Communications Commission, WC Docket No. 02-60 (filed Feb. 28, 2012) (OHN Feb. 28 *Ex Parte* Letter).
Rocky Mountain HealthNet Colorado Health Care Connections	RMHN CHCC	Feb. 28, 2012	Colorado Feb. 28 *Ex Parte* Letter	Letter from George DelGrosso, Rocky Mountain HealthNet, and Steven Summer, Colorado Health Care Connections, to Network, to Christianna Lewis Barnhart, Attorney Advisor, Federal Communications Commission, WC Docket No. 02-60 (filed Feb. 28, 2012) (Colorado Feb. 28 *Ex Parte* Letter).

PARTY	ABBREVIA TION	DATE OF FILING	SHORT CITE	FULL CITE
Pilot Project Group Call (Pennsylvania Mountains Health Care Alliance, Palmetto State Providers Network, North Carolina Telehealth Network, Colorado Health Care Connections, Rocky Mountain HealthNet)	PMHA PSPN NCTN CHCC RMHN	Mar. 13, 2012	Pilot Conference Call Mar. 13 *Ex Parte* Letter (PMHA *et al.*)	Letter from Christianna Lewis Barnhart, Attorney Advisor, Federal Communications Commission, to Marlene H. Dortch, Secretary, Federal Communications Commission, WC Docket No. 02-60 (filed Mar. 13, 2012) (Pilot Conference Call Mar. 13 *Ex Parte* Letter (PMHA *et al.*)).
Universal Service Administrative Company	USAC	Mar. 14, 2012	USAC Observa- tions Letter	Letter from Craig Davis, Vice President, Rural Health Care Division, Universal Service Administrative Company, to Sharon Gillett, Chief, Wireline Competition Bureau, Federal Communications Commission, WC Docket No. 02-60 (filed Mar. 14, 2012) (USAC Observations Letter).
Pilot Project Group Call (Arizona Rural Community Health Information Exchange, Erlanger Health System, Kentucky Behavioral Telehealth Network)	ARCHIE Erlanger KBTN	Mar. 16, 2012	Pilot Conference Call Mar. 16 *Ex Parte* Letter (ARCHIE *et al.*)	Letter from Linda L. Oliver, Attorney Advisor, Federal Communications Commission, to Marlene H. Dortch, Secretary, Federal Communications Commission, WC Docket No. 02-60 (filed Mar. 16, 2012) (Pilot Conference Call Mar. 16 *Ex Parte* Letter (ARCHIE *et al.*)).

PARTY	ABBREVIATION	DATE OF FILING	SHORT CITE	FULL CITE
Universal Service Administrative Company Site Visit Summary (Northeast Ohio Regional Health Information Network, Heartland Unified Broadband Network, PSPN, Iowa Rural Health Telecommunications Program, PMHA)	USAC	Mar. 16, 2012	USAC Mar. 16 Site Visit Reports	Letter from Craig Davis, Vice President, Rural Health Care Division, Universal Service Administrative Company, to Sharon Gillett, Chief, Wireline Competition Bureau, Federal Communications Commission, WC Docket No. 02-60 (filed Mar. 16, 2012) (USAC Mar. 16 Site Visit Reports).
National Association of Rural Health Clinics	NARHC	Mar. 26, 2012	NARHC Mar. 26 *Ex Parte* Letter	Letter from Chin Yoo, Attorney Advisor, Federal Communications Commission, to Marlene H. Dortch, Secretary, Federal Communications Commission, WC Docket No. 02-60 (filed Mar. 26, 2012) (NARHC Mar. 26 *Ex Parte* Letter).
Pilot Project Group Call (Alaska eHealth Network, Southwest Telehealth Access Grid, Tennessee Telehealth Network, Virginia Acute Stroke Telehealth Project, Texas Health Information Network Collaborative)	AEN SWTAG TTN VAST THINC	Mar. 26, 2012	Pilot Conference Call Mar. 26 *Ex Parte* Letter (AEN *et al.*)	Letter from Linda L. Oliver, Attorney Advisor, Federal Communications Commission, to Marlene H. Dortch, Secretary, Federal Communications Commission, WC Docket No. 02-60 (filed Mar. 26, 2012) (Pilot Conference Call Mar. 26 *Ex Parte* Letter (AEN *et al.*)).

PARTY	ABBREVIATION	DATE OF FILING	SHORT CITE	FULL CITE
Pilot Project Group Call (Western New York Rural Area Health Education Center, St. Joseph's Hospital, Sanford Health Collaboration and Communication Channel, Oregon Health Network, Geisinger Health System, Bacon County Health Services, Inc.)	WNYRAHEC St. Joseph's Sanford OHN Geisinger Bacon County	Mar. 26, 2012	Pilot Conference Call Mar. 26 *Ex Parte* Letter (WNYRA HEC *et al.*)	Letter from Linda Oliver, Attorney Advisor, Federal Communications Commission, to Marlene H. Dortch, Secretary, Federal Communications Commission, WC Docket No. 02-60 (filed Mar. 26, 2012) (Pilot Conference Call Mar. 26 *Ex Parte* Letter (WNYRAHEC *et al.*)).
Palmetto State Providers Network	PSPN	Mar. 27, 2012	PSPN Mar. 27 *Ex Parte* Letter	Letter from W. Roger Poston II, Palmetto State Providers Network, to Sharon Gillett, Chief, Wireline Competition Bureau, Federal Communications Commission, WC Docket No. 02-60 (filed Mar. 27, 2012) (PSPN Mar. 27 *Ex Parte* Letter).
National State Offices of Rural Health	NOSORH	Mar. 28, 2012	NOSORH Mar. 28 *Ex Parte* Letter	Letter from Christianna Lewis Barnhart, Attorney Advisor, Federal Communications Commission, to Marlene H. Dortch, Secretary, Federal Communications Commission, WC Docket No. 02-60 (filed Mar. 28, 2012) (NOSORH Mar. 28 *Ex Parte* Letter).
John Gale, Maine Rural Health Research Center	John Gale	Mar. 29, 2012	John Gale Mar. 29 *Ex Parte* Letter	Letter from Linda L. Oliver, Attorney Advisor, Federal Communications Commission, to Marlene H. Dortch, Secretary, Federal Communications Commission, WC Docket No. 02-60 (filed Mar. 29, 2012) (John Gale Mar. 29 *Ex Parte* Letter).

PARTY	ABBREVIATION	DATE OF FILING	SHORT CITE	FULL CITE
Cabarrus Health Alliance	Cabarrus Health Alliance	Apr. 9, 2012	Cabarrus Health Alliance *et al.* Comments	Comments of Cabarrus Health Alliance, Kirby Information Management Consulting, LLC, Microelectronics Center of North Carolina, NC Association of Local Public Health Directors, NC Institute for Public Health, North Carolina Hospital Association, WC Docket No. 02-60 (filed Apr. 9, 2012) (Cabarrus Health Alliance *et al.* Comments)
U.S. Department of Health Information Services, Office of Rural Health Policy	ORHP	Apr. 10, 2012	ORHP Apr. 10 *Ex Parte* Letter	Letter from Christianna Lewis Barnhart, Attorney Advisor, Federal Communications Commission, to Marlene H. Dortch, Secretary, Federal Communications Commission, WC Docket No. 02-60 (filed April 10, 2012) (ORHP Apr. 10 *Ex Parte* Letter).
Universal Service Administrative Company	USAC	Apr. 12, 2012	USAC Needs Assessment	Letter from Craig Davis, Vice President, Rural Health Care Division, Universal Service Administrative Company, to Sharon Gillett, Chief, Wireline Competition Bureau, Federal Communications Commission, WC Docket No. 02-60 (filed Apr. 12 2012) (USAC Needs Assessment).
Universal Service Administrative Company Site Visit Summary (NCTN, Bacon County)	USAC	Apr. 27, 2012	USAC Apr. 27 Site Visit Reports	Letter from Craig Davis, Vice President, Rural Health Care Division, Universal Service Administrative Company, to Sharon Gillett, Chief, Wireline Competition Bureau, WC Docket No. 02-60 (filed Apr. 27, 2012) (USAC Apr. 27 Site Visit Reports).
Universal Service Administrative Company	USAC	May 4, 2012	USAC May 4 Data Letter	Letter from Craig Davis, Vice President, Rural Health Care Division, Universal Service Administrative Company, to Sharon Gillett, Chief, Wireline Competition Bureau, Federal Communications Commission, WC Docket No. 02-60 (filed May 4, 2012) (USAC May 4 Data Letter).

PARTY	ABBREVIATION	DATE OF FILING	SHORT CITE	FULL CITE
Universal Service Administrative Company	USAC	May 30, 2012	USAC May 30 Data Letter	Letter from Craig Davis, Vice President, Rural Health Care Division, Universal Service Administrative Company, to Sharon Gillett, Chief, Wireline Competition Bureau, Federal Communications Commission, WC Docket No. 02-60 (filed May 30, 2012) (USAC May 30 Data Letter).
University of Virginia, VAST Network	UVA	June 8, 2012	UVA June 8 *Ex Parte*	Letter from Elizabeth McCarthy, Attorney Advisor, Federal Communications Commission, to Marlene H. Dortch, Secretary, Federal Communications Commission, WC Docket No. 02-60 (filed June 8, 2012) (UVA June 8 *Ex Parte* Letter).
Universal Service Administrative Company	USAC	June 27, 2012	USAC June 27 Data Letter	Letter from Craig Davis, Vice President, Rural Health Care Division, Universal Service Administrative Company, to Sharon Gillett, Chief, Wireline Competition Bureau, Federal Communications Commission, WC Docket No. 02-60 (filed June 27, 2012) (USAC June 27 Data Letter).
Universal Service Administrative Company	USAC	July 19, 2012	USAC Critical Access Hospitals Report	Letter from Craig Davis, Vice President of Rural Health Care, USAC, to Julie Veach, Chief, WCB, WC Docket No. 02-60 (filed Jul. 19, 2012) (USAC Critical Access Hospitals Report).
Universal Service Administrative Company	USAC	Aug. 2, 2012	USAC Aug. 2 Data Letter	Letter from Craig Davis, Vice President, Rural Health Care Division, Universal Service Administrative Company, to Julie Veach, Chief, Wireline Competition Bureau, Federal Communications Commission, WC Docket No. 02-60 (filed Aug. 2, 2012) (USAC Aug. 2 Data Letter).

PARTY	ABBREVIATION	DATE OF FILING	SHORT CITE	FULL CITE
Universal Service Administrative Company	USAC	Aug. 9, 2012	USAC Aug. 9 Data Letter	Letter from Craig Davis, Vice President, Rural Health Care Division, Universal Service Administrative Company, to Julie Veach, Chief, Wireline Competition Bureau, Federal Communications Commission, WC Docket No. 02-60 (filed Aug. 9, 2012) (USAC Aug. 9 Data Letter).